Deeper Sleep, Richer Life

Sleep Doc's 200 Pearls for Females

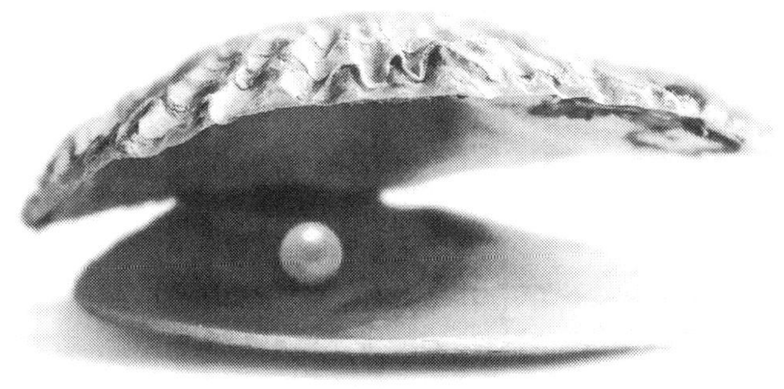

Yatin J. Patel, MD, MBA
Board Certified Sleep Physician
Author, "Sleep Well, Lead Well"

2417 S. Berkshire Drive, Goshen, IN 46526, USA
www.md4lungs.com

The intent of this book and the website is to provide information for educational purposes only. It is also imperative that you speak with your health-care professional before using the information given in this book and on the website. The information provided is not intended to diagnose, treat, cure, or prevent disease.

This book should not be used as a substitute for professional consultation (including detailed history-taking and thorough physical examination) with your physician. The providing of this information does not create a physician-patient relationship, and the owner/author shall not be liable to any person in connection with furnishing this information. We shall have no liability for information provided on this site and in any subsequent exchange. The information provided in this book, and in any subsequent exchange, is intended purely for educational purposes and does not constitute furnishing of medical advice, services, or treatment. The information should not be used to diagnose, treat, or cure a disease process. If you have or suspect you have a medical problem, promptly contact your health-care provider.

None of the statements in this book are an endorsement of any particular product, or a recommendation as to how to treat any particular disease or health-related condition. Yatin J. Patel, MD, shall have no liability as a publisher of information or as a physician or reseller of any products or vendor services, including, without limitation, any liability for defective products. Yatin J. Patel, MD, makes no guarantee or warranty of any kind, expressed, or implied, with respect to (a) the book or (b) products, information, or services displayed in this book.

TO THE FULLEST EXTENT PERMISSIBLE BY APPLICABLE LAW, YATIN J. PATEL, MD, AND HIS SUPPLIERS DISCLAIM ALL WARRANTIES, EXPRESSED OR IMPLIED, INCLUDING, BUT NOT LIMITED TO, IMPLIED WARRANTIES OF TITLE, MERCHANTABILITY, FITNESS FOR PARTICULAR PURPOSE, AND NONINFRINGEMENT. YOU SHOULD NOT USE THE INFORMATION CONTAINED IN THIS BOOK OR ON THE WEBSITE FOR DIAGNOSING A HEALTH PROBLEM OR PRESCRIBING A MEDICATION. YOU SHOULD CAREFULLY READ ALL INFORMATION PROVIDED BY THE MANUFACTURERS OF THE PRODUCTS ON OR IN THE PRODUCT PACKAGING AND LABELS BEFORE USING ANY PRODUCT PURCHASED. YOU SHOULD ALWAYS CONSULT YOUR OWN PHYSICIAN AND MEDICAL ADVISERS.

We are not responsible for the content and performance of recommended books, articles, and websites or for your transactions with them.

If you find this book helpful, please spread the word. Buy additional copies from www.Amazon.com for the women in your life. Profits from the sale of this book support F.E.M.A.L.E. (Food, Education, Medicines, And Love for Everyone) Ashram, a global nonprofit initiative.

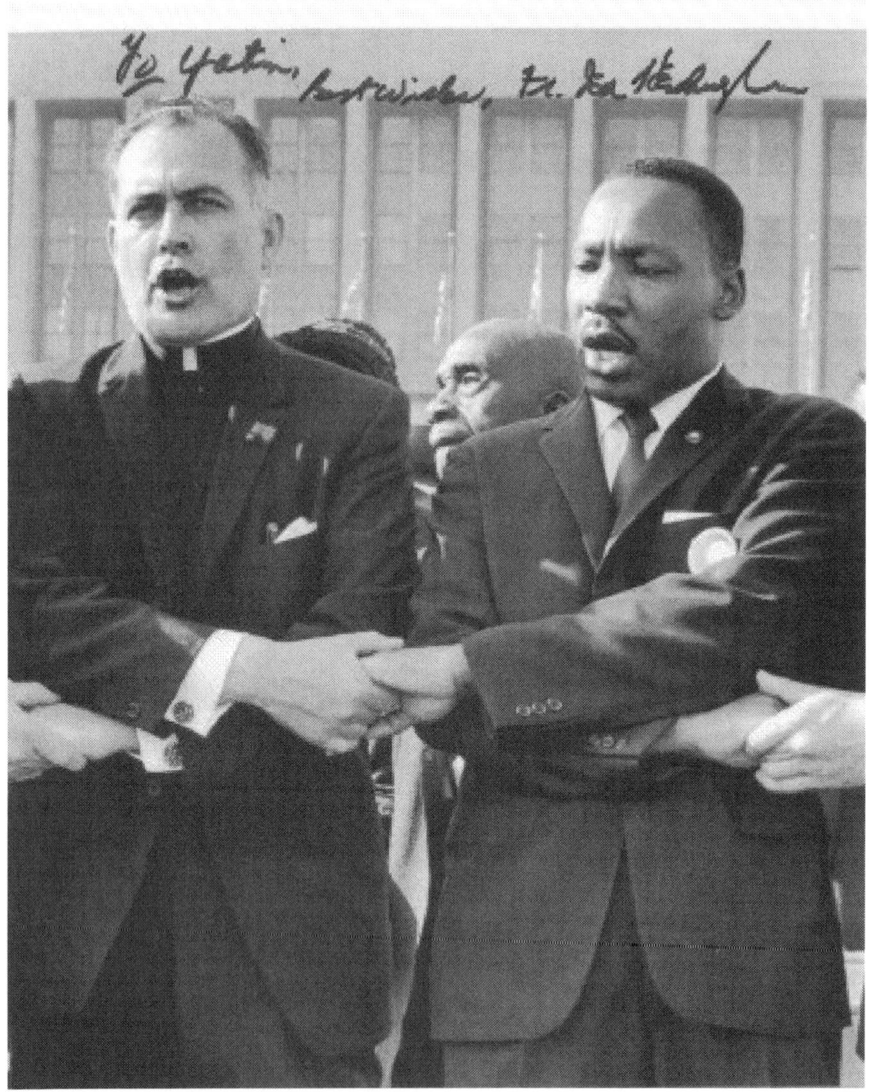

Father Ted Hesburgh (left), whose inspiration and blessings made this book possible

To millions of females who work hard every day despite insufficient sleep

Acknowledgments

During the past twenty years of my clinical practice, I have used the work of medical researchers from around the world for the benefit of my patients, and now I am using it to help you sleep better. Here are a few of them whose lifetime of dedication made this work possible:

Jessica Payne, PhD, University of Notre Dame, Notre Dame, IN

Ralph Downey III, PhD, Loma Linda University, Loma Linda, CA

Matthew P. Walker, PhD, University of California, Berkeley, CA

E. Van der Helm, PhD, and N. Gujar, PhD, University of California, Berkeley, CA

Thomas Roth, PhD, Henry Ford Medical Center, Detroit, MI

William Dement, MD, PhD, and Christian Guilleminault, MD, Stanford University, Stanford, CA

Teofilo L. Lee-Chiong Jr., MD, National Jewish Medical Center, Denver, CO

Thomas J. Balkin, PhD, Walter Reed Army Institute of Research, Bethesda, MD

Nancy J. Wesensten, MD, Walter Reed Army Institute of Research, Bethesda, MD

Sara C. Mednick, MD, University of California, San Diego, CA

Robert Stickgold, MD, Harvard Medical School, Boston, MA

Charles A. Czeisler, MD, PhD, Harvard Medical School, Boston, MA

Diedre Barrett, PhD, Harvard Medical School, Boston, MA

Daniel Goleman, PhD, researcher and author of *Emotional Intelligence*

Matthew A. Wilson, PhD, Massachusetts Institute of Technology, Cambridge, MA

Preface

One of the most powerful women in the business world, Indra Noyi, Time *magazine's top one hundred most influential people in the world, learns on a sunny August day in 2006 that she has been appointed CEO of Pepsi. A flurry of activity follows: meetings after meetings and phone calls after phone calls. Finally, after a long and tiring day, she reaches her home around 10:00 p.m. Her mom quickly congratulates her and asks right away, "Can you run down and get milk? We are out of milk." "Why can't he go?" asks the newly appointed CEO, referring to her husband. "Well, he came in late in the evening. He was tired, so he ate and went to bed. Why can't you go?" her mom persisted.*

You ladies work hard both at home and at work, where you fight male dominance every day. And besides fighting that male dominance in the workplace, you, while shouldering more than your share of family responsibilities, fight insufficient sleep during premenstrual syndrome, menstruation, pregnancy, lactation, menopause, and postmenopause. If you add poor sleep hygiene to this list, what you get is a severely suboptimal life. So, it is of paramount importance that you follow sleep hygiene instructions with fervor and fanaticism.

In this book, I provide the pearls that can help you improve your sleep and thereby regain your life during these unique times. We will first learn sleep physiology and the sleep hygiene instructions, which we all should be following all the time. Then, we shall learn the tips that can help you sleep well during those unique times. Lastly, we will learn how to maximize life when faced with poor sleep secondary to events at home or at work: your daughter's wedding, your mother's emergency surgery, a move into your dream home, your promotion at work, a new product launch, or a major software upgrade at work.

Sleep can be the best investment or the worst one.

You may argue why you can't just drink coffee all day long, enjoy a comfortable sedentary life, doze off for a tempting nap while watching the evening news, work in bed until midnight, watch movies on the laptop while checking e-mails on your iPhone while still in bed (or watch the late-night news on TV and then fall asleep with the TV on), and sleep in on weekends. What is wrong with that?

Remember that you invest one-third of your life in sleep. What are you getting in return? Tiredness? Fatigue? Grumpiness? Achiness? Fogginess? Nervousness? Irritability? How can you change that? How can you maximize the return on your investment? How can you squeeze out maximal life from every waking moment? How can you be maximally alert all day long full of energy, enthusiasm, vigor, and vitality? In the morning, you jump out of bed full of energy as soon as the alarm goes off. At work you walk with a bounce and talk with a smile. You work with boundless energy even in the afternoon. In the evening, you come home still maximally alert and full of energy so that you can play with your kids, enjoy a stimulating conversation with your spouse, read a classic book, listen to your favorite music, and then get ready for bed. Is this really possible? Can we achieve this? Yes, we certainly can. So stop blaming the stress at work or at home and start your journey toward deeper sleep and a richer life.

Over the past twenty years of my clinical practice at the Sneeze & Snooze Clinic and at the IU Health Sleep Center, I have seen thousands of females who improved their life remarkably by improving their sleep. I also believe that for every female I see in the clinic, there are thousands more who can benefit from the tips I shared with those females. Here is my humble attempt at reaching out to those who need help but cannot come to the clinic.

If you follow these tips religiously, then you will fall asleep faster, stay asleep longer, spend more time in deeper stages of sleep, and as a result, wake up refreshed. You will enjoy peak alertness all day long. You will remain happy, cheerful, optimistic, energetic, and enthusiastic all day. You will maximize your problem-solving ability, creativity, big-picture skills, social skills, and spirituality.

You may ask, "What do I do when I can't get a sufficient amount of sleep because of stress at home or at work?" Well, I have been through that, too, from 1989 to 2009. And I can share tips that helped me during those ICU calls that were thirty-six hours and sometimes seventy-two hours long. To make matters worse, I also got poor-quality sleep because I did not practice what I preached. During that vital period, my leadership and my life passed by, which I did not realize at the time. I have combined that unique experience with the latest medical research to come up with a framework that will empower you to regain that lost leadership and life itself. I want you to be better prepared than I was at handling crises both at home and at work, and more important, at enjoying work and cherishing this wonderful gift called life.

Remember that we are here on this beautiful earth for only a finite amount of time. The only way we can squeeze maximum life out of each moment is by maximizing our alertness, even during stressful periods in our lives. I know this is an uphill battle, but with patience, perseverance, practice, and faith, you will learn to enjoy work and life despite unavoidable sleep debt.

Sleep Well, Live Well.

CONTENTS

Section I
Learn Sleep Physiology

Section II
Invest in Sleep Hygiene

- Seek Darkness
- Eliminate Noise
- Stuff a Pillow on His Face
- Try White Noise
- Keep Your Bedroom Cool
- Use the Right Mattress
- Reserve Bedroom for Sleep and Sex Only
- Start Drinking Early
- Stop Smoking
- Eat Light to Sleep Deeply
- Sweat for Sound Sleep
- Run Well, REM Well
- Stay Active at Home and at Work
- Promote REM Sleep with Prayer
- Pray on the Pillow
- Simplify Life for Sound Sleep
- Spend Less, Sleep More

- Practice Specific Pearls to Cure Insomnia
- Conquer Procrastination
- Learn the Benefits of a Power Nap
- Take a Power Nap (Patel's REM nap)
- Learn to Take an Open Eye Nap

Section III

"It's a Female Thing. You Wouldn't Understand."

- Sleep Soundly Despite PMS and Menstruation
- Sleep Well When Sleeping for Two
- Help Baby Sleep through the Night
- Sleep Well during Menopause and Beyond
- Sleep Better Despite Fibromyalgia

Section IV

Insufficient Sleep Leads to Incomplete Life

- Beware of Poor Sleep's Side Effects

- Know Your Sleep Debt
- Regain Your Family Life
- Learn from Politicians' Mistakes
- Get Treated for Obstructive Sleep Apnea
- Eliminate Bad Sleep Habits
- Eliminate Insomnia of Interpersonal Conflict
- Sleep Soundly Even during Excitement
- Eliminate Anxiety about Falling Sleep

Section V

Lead Well Despite Sleep Debt

- Monitor Your Alertness
- Follow the LAMP (Leader's Alertness Maximization Plan)
- Eliminate Midafternoon Madness
- Regain Your Evenings
- Be Happy Despite Sleep Debt
- Collaborate and Create Even When Tired
- Eliminate Irrational Fears
- Control Your Mirror Neurons

- Develop and Use Super Neurons
- Maximize Your Emotional Intelligence
- Remember Poor Sleep Impairs Your IQ
- Manage Information Well
- Use Your Spiritual Strength
- Dream Big Even When Sleepy
- Reverse Ability-Ambition Gap

Concluding Comments

Section I

Sleep Physiology

- Learn about Deep Sleep
- Let REM Sleep Rejuvenate the Leader Within You
- Use REM to Innovate
- Use REM's Crazy Creativity to Transform Your Life
- Know Your Circadian Rhythm
- Go With the Rhythm
- Less Sleep Can't Give You More Life
- Know Your Sleep Number
- Avoid Imitation
- Accept That You Are Not a True Short Sleeper
- Do Not Make Excuses for Insufficient Sleep

o Learn about Deep Sleep

Sleep, an active, organized process, is the restorative and rejuvenating phase of our daily life. It consists of sleep cycles of about ninety minutes each, during which we cycle through light sleep and deep sleep. On a typical night, we go through four to five such cycles, and with each cycle, our REM (rapid eye movement) sleep gets longer, deeper, and more restorative.

The sleep state includes two major types of sleep: REM sleep and non-REM sleep. Non-REM sleep is divided into three different stages, N1, N2, and N3 with stage N3 referred to as "delta sleep." In adults, non-REM sleep accounts for approximately 75 percent of their sleeping time, while REM sleep occupies 25 percent of the normal sleep experience.

Stage N3 and REM sleep play a vital role in memory consolidation, information processing, and retrieval. Adequate duration of deep sleep is necessary to maintain normal levels of cognitive skills such as memory, speech, complex thinking, and creative problem solving.

○ **Let REM Sleep Rejuvenate the Leader within You**

Studies using both MRI and PET technology demonstrate that sleep deprivation diminishes activity in the prefrontal cortex. This area of the brain is responsible for several important functions, including empathy, mood, vision, communication skills, divergent thinking, and problem-solving skills.

The prefrontal cortex, part of the frontal lobe, is the most active area of the brain in rested individuals. However, in sleep-deprived people, this part of the brain nearly shuts down. The majority of the deficits created because of these sleep-deficient shutdowns persist, despite strong individual motivation. The prefrontal cortex governs executive function, which includes our ability to:

- Make sound decisions.
- Behave in a socially acceptable manner; that is, control our urges so as to avoid behavior that is unacceptable or even illegal.
- Plan, discriminate, make decisions, direct and sustain attention while ignoring distractions, and initiate goal-directed behavior.
- Have flexible and innovative thinking and decision making in response to novel and unexpected information and events.

- Integrate emotions and cognition to help resolve ethical dilemmas.

o Remember REM Sleep Leads to Innovation!

REM sleep, the most active state of our existence, has a hyperactive brain in a paralyzed body. Chaotic and incessant neuronal firings characterize REM sleep, leading to tremendous physiological activity and vivid dreams. Devoid of any constraints of time, place, or person, these vivid dreams spark innovation through out-of-the-world thinking. In the process, they help you create a world on your own terms. With a bit of practice, you can tap into this innovative power of your REM sleep.

By using electrodes thinner than our hair, MIT researcher Dr. Matthew Wilson recorded neuronal firing in a rat's brain as the rat ran a maze. He continued this recording when the rat was asleep. To his surprise, he found the neuronal firing during REM sleep was identical to that when the rat was awake and actually running the maze. Interestingly, these neuronal bursts during REM were even more intense than they were during wakefulness.

What's more, while dreaming, we do not respect anatomical barriers. (In fact, the rat would run through the wall.) So, during REM sleep, you are not just thinking outside the box, but also running outside the box without the risk of banging into the wall.

o Use REM to Innovate

Dr. Sara Mednik, a researcher at the University of California, San Diego, administered a remote association test in which she gave participants three words and asked them to come up with a word that would link those three words; for example, given *sixteen*, *heart*, and *candy*, the answer would be *sweet.* After a nap containing REM sleep, participants produced a whopping 40 percent increase in correct answers, which strongly suggests that REM sleep enhanced the formation of associative networks and integration of unassociated information. This was after just a short nap containing REM sleep. Can you imagine the creativity after a full night of sleep containing a total of two hours of REM? Hence, if your teenager presents you with a tough problem, you should say, "Let me REM on it!" I am sure you would wake up with a creative answer that would surprise you and please your teenager. Maybe not, but sleep on a tough problem anyway!

> ***"I think that these dreams involve a search for new and creative ways to put memories and ideas together," said Dr. Robert Stickgold of Harvard Medical School. "They can make associations that we wouldn't make when we're awake."***

Studies have also demonstrated that our mood gets a real boost when we experience adequate amounts of REM sleep. Deprivation of REM sleep, on the other hand, can result in a depressed mood and affect.

- **Know The Historical Evidence Supporting REM Sleep**

Otto Loewi, who received the Nobel Prize in 1938 for his work on the chemical transmission of nerve impulses, wrote:

The night before Easter Sunday of that year I awoke, turned on the light, and jotted down a few notes on a tiny slip of paper. Then I fell asleep again. It occurred to me at 6 AM that during the night I had written down something most important, but I was unable to decipher the scrawl. The next night, at 3 o'clock, the idea returned. It was the design of an experiment to determine whether or not the hypothesis of chemical transmission that I had uttered 17 years ago was correct. I got up immediately, went to the laboratory, and performed a single experiment on a frog's heart according to the nocturnal design.

There have been two Nobel prizes, inventions of numerous medications, and a plethora of very successful stories, novels, and pictures attributed to the crazy creativity of REM sleep.

- **Use REM's Crazy Creativity to Transform Your Life**

Here are a few helpful tips to help you achieve that:

- Accept the fact that we dream every night. We may not remember our dreams, but with training, we can learn to remember and even modify them.
- In the afternoon and in the evening, with positive emotions and unrestrained creativity, intensely contemplate on a major problem.[1] Ask for divine help by praying before retiring to bed. The Bible, in Matthew 18:23–26, says, "Have faith in God. I assure you: If anyone says to this mountain, 'Be lifted up and thrown into the sea,' and does not doubt in his heart, but believes that what he says will happen, it will be done for him." Praying helps us replace negative emotions, which are commonly associated with dreaming, with faith and optimism.
- Keep paper and pencil on your nightstand. When you wake up at night to use the restroom, jot down what you were dreaming about and then go back to bed without thinking further. As soon as your eyes open in the morning, look at your dream notes and elaborate on them.

---

[1] Harvard Medical School researcher Dr. Diedre Barrett has shown that, more than 50 percent of the time, you can dream about what you choose to dream about prior to retiring to bed.

Remember this key point, even if you do not remember your dreams: They do occur every night, and they consolidate your memory and rearrange your information database, helping you think more clearly and, in the process, find a more creative solution.

o Know Your Circadian Rhythm

Chronobiologist Franz Halberg coined the term "circadian," using the Latin *circa* (around) and *diem* or *dies* (day). Its literal meaning is "approximately one day." A person's circadian rhythm is an internal biological clock located in the hypothalamus portion of the brain. It regulates a number of biological, psychological, and behavioral processes over an approximate period of twenty-four hours.

Most of our bodily systems are subject to circadian variations. Bodily systems most affected by circadian variations include the sleep-wake cycle, the system that regulates temperature, heart rate, blood pressure, digestive function, muscle tone, and the endocrine system. The circadian rhythm is responsible for afternoon sleepiness and subsequent propensity for serious error and significant decline in our executive function. This afternoon dip in alertness is deeper and more prolonged in the presence of sleep debt.

○ Go with the Rhythm

Use the might of Mother Nature to your advantage. Going against Mother Nature by ignoring circadian rhythm will shorten your deep sleep (stage N3 and REM sleep). Always maintain a consistent time to rise, even when circumstances prevent you from going to bed at your normal time. And, yes, that includes weekends. There is no point in going to bed two hours late on weekends and waking up two hours late the next day. There is no net gain. In fact, there is a net loss, because it disrupts your intrinsic rhythm, the sole cause of reduced productivity on Monday mornings.

o Less Sleep Can't Give You More Life

As a busy female, you may ask, "Can I invest less and make more?" It is a perfectly legitimate question. Van Dongen and others studied participants after four, six, and eight hours of sleep for fourteen days and found a significant dose-dependent decline in their neurocognitive performance. Belenky, Dinges, and other researchers have also reported similar findings.

In short, you certainly can achieve more by sleeping less, but at a significant health, cognitive, and behavioral cost. Thus, by sleeping less, you can read more, but you will remember less. You can check more e-mails, but your responses may not reflect your true leadership skills. You can interact with more people, but you might be less perceptive. You can work on more problems, but your solutions might be less creative. You can make more decisions, but they may not be correct ones. In short, if you are sleeping less, you might be a liability, as opposed to an asset.

o Know Your Sleep Number

The need for sleep varies considerably among individuals. The average desirable sleep length is between seven hours and eight and a half hours per day.[2] For you, it could be seven hours. For your spouse, it could be eight and a half hours. As a general rule, whatever sleep length you need to feel maximally alert for sixteen hours all day the next day is the amount of sleep your brain needs to function at peak potential.

o Avoid Imitation

My wife needs seven hours of sleep, but I need eight. Your chief financial officer (CFO) may need seven and a half hours of sleep, while you may need eight and a half to function at your peak potential.

Do not try to imitate when it comes to sleep duration. Your brain is unique, and you need to give it as much or as little sleep as it needs to perform at peak all day long.

---

[2] Although most people need seven to nine hours of sleep each night to function well the next day, the National Sleep Foundation (NSF) Women and Sleep poll found that the average woman aged thirty to sixty sleeps only six hours and forty-one minutes during the workweek.

o Accept That You Are Not a True Short Sleeper

Based on a study done by Dr. Ying-Hui Fu and his team at the University of California, San Francisco, the short sleeper gene, a rare mutation, is present in only 3 percent of the population. And the majority of our leaders get less than six hours of sleep, certainly during stressful periods in their professional or personal lives. Dr. Ying-Hui Fu commented that while these people sleep less, we do not know if they need less sleep. We do not yet know if short sleepers have increased long-term morbidity and mortality.

Researchers have also found that these short-sleepers fall asleep faster on a multiple sleep latency test (MSLT). In this test, subjects are asked to take five daytime naps, two hours apart. On average, a person who is not excessively sleepy will fall asleep in fifteen minutes. These short-sleepers fell asleep in less than ten minutes, a few even in less than five minutes, indicating their abnormal daytime sleepiness.[3] It has also been observed that these short sleepers take unplanned naps in or between meetings, while traveling, and even at public gatherings.[4]

---

[3] Pepsi's CEO Indra Nooyi prides herself in sleeping only four hours every night. I would love to prove that she is excessively sleepy, by doing an MSLT in my sleep lab.

[4] President Clinton was caught napping at the inauguration of the Clinton Public Library in his home state. On another occasion, at an event honoring Dr. Martin Luther King Jr. at Convent Avenue Baptist Church

"Sleep is for the weak, Mr. President," Secretary of Defense Robert McNamara to President John F. Kennedy during the Cuban Missile Crisis

in Harlem, the former president was also caught nodding off.

o Do Not Make Excuses for Insufficient Sleep

My overworked colleagues, unaware of the research cited above, also continue to argue against sufficient sleep. Here is a list of arguments made by skeptics of sufficient sleep and my responses:

- *I don't need eight hours of sleep.* Studies have shown that restricting sleep to four or six hours (compared to eight hours) for fourteen days causes a dose-dependent decline in neurocognitive performance.
- *I only need five hours of sleep.* The short-sleeper gene, a rare mutation, is present in only 3 percent of the population (Ying-Hui Fu, University of California, San Francisco). The majority of leaders get less than six hours of sleep, certainly during a major event or catastrophe.
- *I can fight sleep deprivation with strong motivation.* Motivation improves attention but not creativity, flexibility, mood, perception, and information management.
- *I have achieved a lot by sleeping less.* You could achieve even more by working on your alertness intelligence.

- *I don't perceive the deficit in my performance.* Sleep deprivation adversely affects prefrontal cortex (the executive center), which is essential for successful self-evaluation. This makes us unaware of our deficit.
- *I am highly productive.* You have increased your output as a worker/manager, at the expense of executive output.
- *The stakes are so high that sleep has to be on the back burner.* This is exactly the reason you should be giving sleep a top priority. Also, there are alertness-maximization techniques (discussed in sections II and III) that can help you.
- *I don't want to sleep away a third of my life.* Investment in sleep will enrich your life qualitatively, both at home and at work.
- *I will sleep when I am dead.* Unfortunately, studies have shown increased mortality associated with insufficient sleep. You must sleep eight hours every night if you want a successful career that can span five to six decades.

Sleep is a process of the brain, for the brain, and by the brain.

In this section, we learned about various sleep stages, the sleep architecture, the circadian rhythm, and sleep duration. In the next section, we will learn about the sleep habits that can help us maximize deep sleep and thereby life.

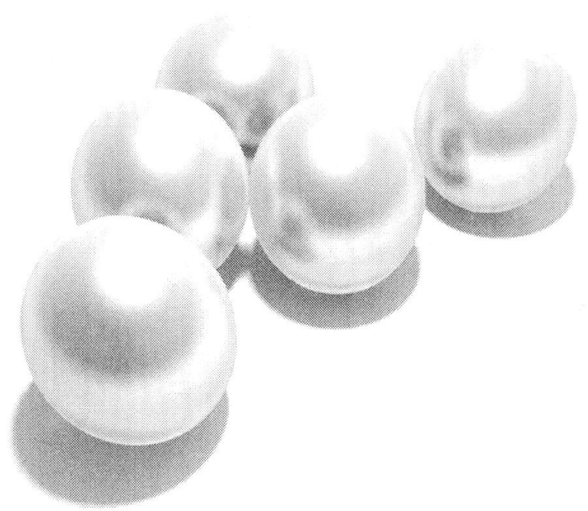

Section II
Invest in Sleep Hygiene

- Seek Darkness
- Eliminate Noise
- Stuff a Pillow on His Face
- Try White Noise
- Keep Your Bedroom Cool
- Use the Right Mattress
- Reserve Bedroom for Sleep and Sex Only
- Start Drinking Early
- Stop Smoking
- Eat Light to Sleep Deeply
- Sweat for Sound Sleep
- Run Well, REM Well
- Stay Active at Home and at Work
- Promote REM Sleep with Prayer
- Pray on the Pillow

- **Simplify Life for Sound Sleep**
- **Spend Less, Sleep More**
- **Practice Specific Pearls to Cure Insomnia**
- **Conquer Procrastination**
- **Learn the Benefits of a Power Nap**
- **Take a Power Nap (Patel's REM nap)**
- **Learn to Take an Open Eye Nap**

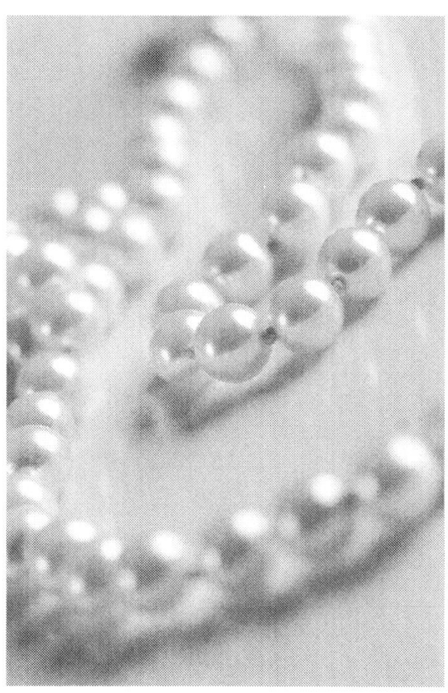

Sleep doesn't differentiate us from animals, but sleep hygiene does.[5] And what is sleep hygiene?

Sleep hygiene is your personal set of habits that determines the quality of your sleep. Sleep hygiene helps you stay healthy by keeping your brain (most important, the executive center) and your body rested and strong. With poor sleep hygiene, you are not only getting insufficient sleep, but also poor-quality sleep. In order to get the most return on your investment in sleep, you must follow sleep hygiene fanatically.

Unfortunately, poor sleep hygiene is endemic. Most of us stay up too late and get up too early. We often overstimulate ourselves by working late into the evening and then watching television in bed. We may even use alcohol, thinking it will give us a better night's sleep. But alcohol, even though it puts us to sleep, causes frequent arousals and thereby robs us of deeper stages of sleep.

---

[5] Michael Bonsignore regards sleep as a necessary evil or sunk cost, while Warren Buffet looks at sleep as the best investment one can make.

Create a Sanctuary for Sleep

You spend one-third of your life in your bedroom. Well, if you pay attention and modify your bedroom by following these simple tips, you will fall asleep faster, stay asleep longer, spend more time in restorative stages (N3 and REM) of sleep and wake up refreshed every morning.

- **Seek Darkness**

The pineal gland, a tiny structure located at the base of the brain, secretes melatonin, a powerful sleep-promoting agent. Based on our internal rhythm, this secretion starts in the evening approximately two hours prior to sleep onset and peaks two hours prior to wakefulness. This whole process leading to melatonin secretion is extremely sensitive to bright light. Light emanating from even a tiny phone screen can reduce this secretion and prevent you from falling asleep and getting enough deep sleep. Here are a few tips to help you maximize your internal melatonin secretion.

- Choose dark drapes or blinds for the bedroom windows. You can also apply black film over glass windows to block out light completely. A dim night-light to guide you safely to the restroom at night is acceptable as long as you are not facing it in your favorite sleeping position. Also, choose a night-light with the lowest brightness. Ideally, the bedroom should be so dark that you should not be able to see your outstretched hand!
- Turn the alarm clock away and keep the brightness to a minimum. My personal preference is not to keep the clock in the bedroom at all.
- Completely turn off all the electronic devices including stereo, satellite boxes, TV, laptop, iPad, and others. Again my preference, as we have discussed before, is not to have these devices in the bedroom at all. If you use them in the evening, please use them outside the bedroom and with lowest possible brightness to maximize melatonin secretion.
- Sport those cool-looking designer sunglasses while driving home in the evening or during outdoor activities in the backyard. Your pineal gland will love you for that.

Remember that melatonin is an ally, while light is an enemy.

- **Eliminate Noise**

Your bedroom should be a quiet place. Not only can noise prevent you from falling asleep, it can repeatedly awaken you at night and keep you from getting the restorative sleep you need. There are patients who tell me that they can fall asleep and stay asleep even if bombs are falling, but the fact remains that the noise, too faint to be noticed, can cause microarousals (several seconds of wakefulness like activity on EEG) and thereby lighten the sleep stage. We see this in our sleep lab when a patient is exposed to a sudden noise of any kind.

- **Stuff a Pillow on His Face (Just Kidding!)**

Snoring occurs from the vibration of the soft tissue caused by air trying to go through a narrow upper airway. When this airway shuts off repeatedly at night, it is called obstructive sleep apnea. Obstructive sleep apnea, a serious and potentially fatal disorder, affects approximately 10 percent of the adult population. Snoring, daytime fatigue, witnessed apnea (cessation of respiration for more than ten seconds), morning headaches, dry throat, and waking up gasping for air are common features of this disorder, which is being increasingly recognized as a formidable enemy of corporate America. Read more about this disorder later on in this book.

Snoring even in the absence of sleep apnea can cause these microarousals, which can prevent you from spending enough time in deep stages of sleep. First and foremost, fill out the STOP questionnaire to make sure you do not have sleep apnea. If you do not have fatigue, tiredness, excessive sleepiness, impaired cognition, high blood pressure, or witnessed apnea (pauses in your breathing during sleep), then you have simple snoring. The following tips can help minimize snoring.

- Weight loss can help snoring by reducing the amount of fat deposition around the upper airway. It also helps tighten the upper airway muscles, which keep the airway open during sleep.
- Alcohol relaxes upper airway muscles, narrows its lumen, and makes snoring worse. It can even turn benign snoring into obstructive sleep apnea. Avoid it religiously within three hours of bedtime. This is easier than you think. Start drinking at five, stop at seven, and go to bed at ten. A perfect evening!
- Avoid sleeping on your back. In some patients, sleeping on the back makes the snoring worse as it causes the large tongue and the fat in front of the neck to fall on the upper airway thereby narrowing it. Avoid sleeping on your back by using positional therapy. Take a tennis ball, put it in an old sock, and sew that sock on the back of an extra nightshirt such that this tennis ball will be on your spine between your shoulder blades. The discomfort of the tennis ball will force you away from sleeping on the back. Try it. It is not cool, but it does work. If one tennis ball does not do the trick, try two!

- Talk to your dentist about your snoring. A customized oral appliance can help eliminate snoring or even mild obstructive sleep apnea. This denture-like device keeps the lower jaw forward, maintains the tone of the upper airway muscles, and prevents upper airway closure during sleep. While the American Academy of Sleep Medicine recommends such customized and adjustable devices, it does not recommend the nonadjustable and noncustomized oral appliances you may find on the Web.
- Try Breathe Right strips. You may find them helpful especially if you suffer from nasal stuffiness or obstruction.
- Talk to your doctor about allergy testing to rule out nasal allergies. Your doctor can also prescribe you nasal steroid spray, which can help reduce nasal inflammation, bogginess, and narrowing.

- **Try White Noise**

Soothing white noise can help promote deep sleep. Based on your preference, you can use the sounds of ocean, nature, or running water to achieve a similar effect. Dr. Spencer and his colleagues at Queen Charlotte's Hospital in London studied two groups of twenty neonates, between two and seven days old, in a randomized trial. Sixteen (80 percent) fell asleep within five minutes in response to white noise compared with only five (25 percent) who fell asleep spontaneously in the control group. White noise may help mothers settle difficult babies.

If you want to use white noise for sleep induction, please check out www.simplynoise.com. I found their downloadable mp3 sound track immensely soothing and helpful. You can also download its smartphone app for 99 cents. I recommend white noise especially to patients who prefer to sleep with their TV on.

- **Keep Your Bedroom Cool**

Bats sleep sixteen hours a day because they are in cool, dark caves. We, too, fall sleep faster and stay asleep longer in cool temperatures. Our core body temperature has a circadian rhythm with the peak temperature occurring in the evening and the lowest one occurring in the early morning hours when REM sleep is longest and deepest. The fall of core body temperature in late evening facilitates sleep onset, while persistence of lower core body temperature promotes deep sleep and longer sleep duration. A study by Dr. Parker and colleagues at Emory University in Atlanta, Georgia, showed that lowering the temperature of dialysis fluid from 37°C to 35°C improved sleep quality in patients on long-term dialysis. These patients fell asleep quicker, went into REM sleep faster, and stayed asleep longer.

- **Walls Can Help Too**

Use darker colors on the wall. Hang relaxing pictures of beautiful landscapes, gorgeous mountains, Buddha meditating, or the baby Jesus sleeping in his mother's lap. You can buy such posters quite inexpensively at www.allposters.com, or, better yet, use your own travel photos to add a personal touch to your bedroom walls.

- **Use the Right Mattress**

  Arya Nick Shamie, MD, associate professor of orthopedic surgery and neurosurgery at Santa Monica UCLA Medical Center, emphasizes that the mattress needs to support your body in a neutral position, one in which your spine has a nice curvature and your buttocks, heels, shoulders, and head are supported in proper alignment. "If the mattress is too firm, it will push on those main pressure points and take you out of alignment," Shamie told WebMD. "If it's too soft, those pressure points won't be properly supported, so your whole body flops back." Both of these scenarios can lead to an achy morning. Researchers in Spain who studied people with long-term back pain found that, on a 10-point hard-to-soft scale, people who slept on a medium-to-firm mattress (5.6 on the scale) had less back pain than those who slept on a softer mattress. But, what if you like a firm mattress and your spouse prefers a soft one? Take your spouse to a Sleep Number mattress store during a quiet afternoon and take a relaxing nap to find out for yourself! I suggest trying number 80 on one half and number 40 on the other half.

Research temperature-controlled mattresses, Posturepedic mattresses, or other such high-tech mattresses and choose the one that suits you. You can also explore power-adjusted bed frames, especially if you suffer from back pain, knee pain, or acid reflux. I found this article on WebMD immensely helpful in choosing the right mattress: http://www.webmd.com/sleep-disorders/features/how-to-pick-your-perfect-mattress.

- **Reserve Bedroom for Sex and Sleep Only**[6]

Work-related activities will result in a state of hyperarousal, which will delay sleep onset and, more important, rob you of your deep (stage N3 and REM) sleep. Hence, do not take Excel spreadsheets and PowerPoint presentations to bed. Do not check e-mails or text messages in the bedroom. Is this rule difficult to follow? Yes, but not impossible. And if you want to get the maximum amount of rest from the limited hours of sleep, you have to follow this rule. Start by working in the living room or study before finally retiring to your bedroom. Make this a habit. Seek your family's cooperation in this and you will improve their sleep too!

---

[6] Several years ago, I was giving a talk to a group of nurses, and the slide read, "Use bed only for sleep." A naughty nurse reacted, "Where do we do the *other* thing?" Hence the modification!

o Start Drinking Early

Recognize that alcohol induces sleep, but it also causes poor-quality sleep marked by frequent arousals, leading to a lighter sleep at the expense of REM sleep. Alcohol further disrupts sleep by making snoring and sleep apnea. It also disrupts sleep by increasing the frequency of nighttime urination. In *Macbeth*, Shakespeare wrote, "It provoketh and unprovoketh." He was referring to the fact that alcohol provokes sexual desire but retards sexual performance. Similarly, alcohol induces sleep but robs you of your deep sleep. Because of this, the general recommendation in sleep-medicine practice is to avoid consuming alcohol six hours before bedtime. I try to be nice to my friends and request they avoid it within three hours of bedtime. This still did not go well with some of my friends, hence I changed the message to, "Start drinking early," and now they love the message and the messenger! As stated earlier, you can start enjoying alcohol at five, stop drinking at seven, and go to bed at ten. A perfect evening!

Absolutely avoid alcohol within six hours of bedtime while going through insomnia treatment. For patients not suffering from insomnia, the recommendation is to avoid alcohol within three hours of bedtime. Alcohol increases the number of microarousals (wakefulness activity of ten seconds or longer on an EEG recording) during sleep, robs you of your deep sleep, and makes your sleep nonrestorative. It also causes adrenaline overstimulation when the alcohol level in the blood is coming down.

- **Stop Smoking**

Make every effort to quit smoking completely, because it affects your sleep too. Nicotine is a stimulant that robs you of your deep sleep. My patients have had great success using faith and the support of their family. Talk to your doctor about nicotine patch and gum and other medications that can help. You can also try calling 1-800-QUIT-NOW or visiting www.BecomeAnEx.org, an online support program from the Mayo Clinic that my patients have used successfully. Both of these services are free. But even after all of these you cannot quit, certainly avoid smoking within three hours of your bedtime.

o Eat Light to Sleep Deeply

Avoid eating a heavy meal before bedtime; the process of digestion interferes with falling asleep and may reduce the amount of deep sleep. It also exacerbates acid reflux, which can further compound your sleep problems. Bedtime milk and cookies, however, can help you fall asleep as milk contains tryptophan, a naturally occurring sleep-promoting substance.

o Sweat for Sound Sleep

In ancient times, the harder one worked, the better one slept because of the physical nature of the work. Today, however, your work, unfortunately, does not lead to better sleep because it is emotionally and intellectually, but not physically, demanding. This is where exercise comes into play. Regularly exercising, even for twenty minutes a day, has been shown to improve sleep architecture. Not only does it make you fall asleep quicker, but it also increases the duration of deep sleep and thus makes your sleep immensely more restorative. Exercising has such comprehensive health and performance benefits that it has become my personal favorite of all sleep-hygiene instructions. Please make every effort possible to incorporate exercise in your daily routine—it will help you enjoy life to the fullest!

- **Choose to Exercise**

My patients often complain they don't have time for exercise because their daily schedules simply will not allow it. But exercise is a matter of choice, not time. Remember, we are all given the same amount of time: twenty-four hours a day, seven days a week. How you choose to spend your time can mean the difference between success and failure.

- **Work Out to De-stress**

Stress makes it difficult to fall asleep and even more difficult to get an adequate amount of N3 and REM sleep, where we get physical, mental, emotional, and spiritual rest. How do we deal with this stress? Some use alcohol or prescription drugs to help manage their stressful lives. But even these are little more than futile Band-Aid attempts at solving the real problem, and if alcohol or prescription drugs are misused, they can create an even larger problem.

A lot of my patients claim they are too stressed to work out. In fact, most are too stressed not to exercise. Focus and balance are needed when it comes to executive tasks such as goal setting, problem solving, communication, and team building. Exercise releases hormones that help you relax and bring focus back into your life. Exercise is a natural remedy that brings the body into a state of balance.

Following are some additional ways that exercise will de-stress your life:

- Exercise provides you with a mini-vacation that lets you escape from the stressors and pressures of the day. It gives you a period of solitude, when you can recharge your battery while contemplating important matters that need your attention. It can also be a time for creative thinking and problem solving.

- Exercise detoxifies. Psychosocial stressors cause a significant number of biochemical reactions in the human body. The fight-or-flight response brought about by stress causes the cardiovascular system to accelerate and the gastrointestinal system to slow down. In addition, certain neurotransmitters are activated, hormones are released, and nutrition is metabolized. Exercise detoxifies the body by eliminating the fight-or-flight response, thus allowing the body to return to homeostasis.
- Exercise releases endorphins, a naturally occurring morphine-like substance that provides pain control and euphoria while enhancing N3 and REM sleep. Negative emotions, such as fear and anger, whether expressed or repressed, play a major role in the progression of disease. Several notable research studies confirm this often-forgotten fact. Exercise offers a positive way to release the caustic energy of anger. It provides a healthy catharsis that allows you to dodge the otherwise devastating effects that anger can have on your physical well-being.
- Exercise boosts the immune system. The simple fact is, when fit people are injured or become ill, they recover faster because their immune system is stronger.

- Exercise makes you fall asleep faster. It also improves sleep architecture and makes sleep more restorative by increasing the percentage of N3 and REM sleep. A short twenty-minute investment in exercise will improve your deep sleep so much that you will end up recouping that investment and more.
- Exercise leads to sustainable excellence both at home and at work. Exercise also reduces your risk of an early death. Regular exercise improves your health by lowering the risk of developing high blood pressure, heart disease, diabetes, colon cancer, and depression. Regular exercise helps you control your weight while building healthy muscles, bones, and joints. It also reduces your risk of falling. A regular exercise program doesn't need to be a grueling experience, nor does it need to be time-consuming. You will experience excellent results through as little as twenty-five minutes of strength training and thirty minutes of aerobic training twice per week. And the benefits will far outweigh the time invested.

Consider our ancestors. They did not have the health problems that accompany a sedentary lifestyle. To provide for themselves and their families, they had to work hard physically. As a result, they stayed strong and healthy. Today we lead sedentary lives that don't require much physical work, such as chopping, planting, tilling, harvesting, digging, and similar daily work activities. During our working hours, many of us sit at computers and monitor various aspects of our employer's business or our own. At home, we occupy ourselves with television, video games, the Internet, and other computer-based activities that do not require much movement. We need to get out of our seats and get moving. We need to rediscover the joy of an active and healthy lifestyle. If we do not, then disaster is waiting to happen.

- **Run Well, REM Well**

The American College of Sports Medicine defines aerobic exercise as "any activity that uses large muscle groups, can be maintained continuously, and is rhythmic in nature." An aerobic exercise overloads the heart and lungs, causing them to work harder than when at rest.

Many people think aerobic exercise only involves dance. While aerobic dance is a great way to exercise, other aerobic exercises are just as effective. These include swimming, stair climbing, running, jumping rope, fitness walking, in-line skating, cross-country skiing, and bicycling.

By using aerobic exercise to keep your heart rate elevated for a continuous period, you begin moving to a much healthier life.

- **Stay Active at Home and at Work**

If you're feeling too busy to work out, here are a few practical tips to help. You can find your own too.

- Go from bed to bike in the morning. As soon as the alarm goes off, get on the stationary bike, and then check your e-mails and plan your day. Read your industry journal while pedaling the bike. You can buy laptop stands[7] that work well with bikes and even treadmills.
- Take the stairs during breaks. It will get your blood flowing, heart pumping, and mind going. We have hospital colleagues who walk in the basement of the hospital during lunch break regularly.
- Meet in the gym instead of the boardroom. Paddle a stationary bike instead of sitting in the chair during staff meetings.
- Take a hike. Instead of meeting your production supervisor in the office, walk the floor of the factory. If you walk fast enough, you can get a good twenty-minute workout and also meet workers who would appreciate seeing your face.

---

[7] The Web site www.airdesks.com has nice-looking, functional, and affordable laptop stands.

- Play at noon. We used to have a racquetball league at the hospital where physicians would get together during their lunch break to play racquetball. This annihilates the midafternoon sleepiness, maximizes alertness, and improves executive output by at least 30 percent, in addition to destroying disastrous decision making.

Please talk to your doctor before you begin any kind of physical exercise program. Share the kinds of exercise you're planning to do, as well as your outcome goals. Ask your doctor if your target heart rate calculation is appropriate for you and if there are any medical tests you need to complete before starting an exercise schedule.

o Promote REM Sleep with Prayer

Busy executives from companies all across the United States believe in the power of prayer. Leaders who have strong faith find it easier to meet challenges and overcome any obstacles that appear in their path. Plus, people who pray, especially before going to bed at night, tend to get a better night's sleep than people who don't. Prayer replaces toxic emotions with positive ones that are amplified during REM sleep, so you wake up in the morning with enthusiasm, energy, and optimism. If that's not enough to get you to your knees, what will it take?

o Prayer Provides Personal Growth

In the Company of Prayer is an e-mail subscription service[8] created specifically for business executives. Through its Morning Briefing service, it delivers concise devotionals to the in-boxes of its subscribers each workday. Executive Editor Leslie Blanco says, "As workdays grow longer, time for personal growth, including in the area of spirituality, necessarily overlaps with the business agenda. A daily prayer prompt

[8] You can subscribe to this service at www.companyofprayer.com.

appeals to these executives who also appreciate simply being reminded they are in the company with others who share their emphasis on faith."

Morning Briefing subscribers really enjoy reading the daily e-mail devotions. Tim LeVecke, CEO of LeVecke Corporation, a bottler and marketer of distilled spirits, is one such subscriber. "The Morning Briefing is the first e-mail I open each day because it provides an opportunity for a moment of personal focus and reflection that carries me throughout the day," LeVecke said.

The apostle Paul said we are to pray without ceasing. He also said we are to rejoice in the Lord always. That pretty much covers everything, but some biblical examples offer a little more insight. Daniel had the discipline of prayer firmly entrenched in his life, so much so that it cost him a trip to the lion's den. David started each day with his requests, anticipating God's answers so he could praise God at the close of the day. Jesus got up before the sun rose and went off by himself to pray. And the believers prayed when there was a need.

- **Pray on the Pillow**

From a sleep and leadership standpoint, praying on the pillow (before sleep, after sleep, and at afternoon naps), along with on-the-go one-line prayers, works the best. Praying before sleep eliminates negative emotions. Praying after sleep prepares you for the day. It infuses energy, enthusiasm, and optimism. Praying with your afternoon nap recharges your spiritual engine, while on-the-go prayers maintain your optimism during the challenges at work.

Prayer should be both a discipline that we exercise daily and a free flow of communication with God about whatever concerns us. Pray when you are stumped by a word or phrase, when you are up against a deadline, before signing a contract, and when turning in a manuscript. God's mercies are new every morning, so no matter how bad yesterday was, today is truly a new day in his kingdom.

Here are a few of my favorite prayers.

- ***As I dream tonight, my Lord, take me to the enchanted corners of every galaxy.***
- ***As I sleep, my Lord, replace hatred from my subconscious with faith and love.***

- *As I sleep, Lord, fill up my vast subconscious with hope, happiness, joy, and bliss. And then wake me up with the highest level of consciousness.*
- *Help me serve humanity with unshakable faith, empathy, and enthusiasm.*
- *Help me enjoy every moment today.*
- *Be my energy today.*
- *Give me the strength to carry on.*
- *Instill, in my brain, noble thoughts from every direction.*
- *Keep me polite amid impolite, considerate amid inconsiderate, happy amid unhappy, and optimistic amid pessimistic today.*

- **Simplify Life for Sound Sleep.**

Our finance professor at Notre Dame used to ask, "Do you want to sleep well or eat well?" He was referring to the money earned at the expense of sleep. You can't get sufficient duration of sound sleep if you are stretching yourself too thin trying to earn more and more. You have to find that elusive balance between "eating well and sleeping well." Money earned at the expense of sleep, health, and family time cannot bring you happiness.

- **Spend Less, Sleep More**

Disciplined personal finances will help your journey toward sound sleep, perfect health, and a balanced life. Make an effort to keep in touch with your friends and colleagues who practice simple living and high thinking. Frequently visit the website www.zenhabits.net to help moderate your urge to spend lavishly. Happiness does not come from owning, but from doing and giving. Self-indulgence that ties you up in a career you don't want is a noose around your neck. Solicit your spouse's and children's cooperation in your quest for a balanced life. They are your closest allies and strongest supporters. You will be amazed at how much cooperation you get when you patiently discuss your passion and demonstrate self-restraint, discipline, and willpower.

This may not happen overnight, but with love, faith, and persistence, you will receive the cooperation and support of your loved ones.

- **Practice These Specific Pearls If You Suffer from Insomnia[9]**

The vast majority of patients with insomnia have a brain that has difficulty relaxing, hence it is of paramount importance that they help themselves by following sleep hygiene instructions religiously. Here are a few pearls for those suffering from insomnia.

[9] A National Sleep Foundation's Sleep in America poll revealed that women are more likely than men to have difficulty falling and staying asleep and to experience more daytime sleepiness at least a few nights/days a week.

- **Trust Mother Nature.**

Remember also that sleep is a normal physiological phenomenon. You do not have to do anything to get it! By following the above tips, we are simply making sure that we do not fight Mother Nature. We are undoing some of the bad habits we have acquired over the years. Follow these tips to get the maximum amount of deepest sleep, but do not worry about it—as this anxiety can be counterproductive. There is a story of a king in ancient India who suffered from sleep difficulties. He ordered his soldier to bring in the best physician in the continent. "I will behead you if you don't find an answer to my sleep problem," he shouted. Poor physician thought about this for a second or so and then replied, "I can prepare the best sleeping remedy known to mankind, but I need a week to make this special medicine, Your Highness." A week later, he walked into the palace, met the king, opened his bag, got a bottle out, and instructed the king to take a spoonful of this precious medicine at bedtime with one condition. "If you think of the camel after taking it, this medicine loses its effectiveness and will not work." The king was excited and delighted, took this medicine, but kept on thinking about the camel and could not sleep. Night after night, he got more and more tired of this whole ordeal. One evening he threw the medicine bottle away, rode the camel, came home, played with his son, retired to bed free of anxiety and slept like a baby!

- **Pray on the pillow.**

This is especially important for patients suffering from insomnia. REM sleep is a powerful amplifier of emotions, especially negative ones such as fear, anxiety, hatred, and anger. To use this amplifier to your advantage, you need to focus on positive emotions all day and then, at bedtime, purge your mind of whatever negative emotions it has collected all day. This is where even a short prayer comes into the picture. Remember, faith drives away fear.

- **Do not carry a grudge to bed with you.** Bedtime is not the time to review your anger against others who have hurt you in some way. Luke 6:27–29 in the Bible says it best: "But I say to you who listen: Love your enemies, do good to those who hate you, bless those who curse you, pray for those who mistreat you. If anyone hits you on the cheek, offer the other also." Forgiveness always brings peace, and there is no better sleep aid than a soul at peace. Forgive yourself; forgive others.
- **Learn a relaxing bedtime routine.** A warm shower can help, because cooling off after a shower can be conducive to sleep. Listening to soothing music can calm your anxious nerves. A glass of skim milk and cookies can also help, because milk contains tryptophan, a naturally occurring sleep-promoting agent.
- **Go to bed only when sleepy, not just tired.** Read a relaxing book. Listen to soothing and calming music.
- **If you are not asleep after approximately twenty minutes[10], get out of bed.** This will prevent formation of learned insomnia. Do something relaxing in the living room. Return to bed only when sleepy.

[10] Get out of bed when you get frustrated about not being able to sleep. This may happen at 15 min or at 30 min.

- **Keep the clock face turned away.** Looking at a clock at night will stimulate your brain.
- **Don't fight Mother Nature**. Even on weekends and even after a bad night, get up at the same time every morning. Use your built-in circadian rhythm to your advantage in this fight against insomnia.
- **Avoid taking naps** while going through insomnia treatment. If you must take a nap for emergency purposes, follow the two-twenty rule of napping. Do not nap after two o'clock, and do not nap for longer than twenty minutes. A ten- to fifteen-minute power nap in the early afternoon can energize your day and give you two days in one. But even a brief ten-minute nap in the evening will make it difficult for you to fall asleep and stay asleep, and it will rob you of your deep sleep that night.
- **Use your bed only for sleep and sex.** Ignore your laptop or smartphone completely when in bed. When working on your laptop in the evening, keep the screen brightness to a minimum.[11] Watching TV in bed will stimulate your brain too. Get rid of the TV in the bedroom.

---

[11] As mentioned earlier, bright light inhibits melatonin secretion from your internal pacemaker. This will make it difficult to fall asleep.

- **Recognize that exercise is the best ally of sound sleep**. It helps us fall asleep quickly, stay asleep longer, and get more REM sleep. Even after a rough night, get twenty to thirty minutes of exercise any time during the day, as long as it is not just before retiring to bed.
- **Do not eat a big meal just before bedtime.** The digestion process and acid reflux will both interfere with sleep.

o **Avoid caffeine.** Caffeine has a twenty-four-hour duration of action, so a cup of coffee consumed at seven in the morning is still in your bloodstream at ten at night when you are trying to fall asleep. To avoid caffeine withdrawal, please taper off caffeine over several weeks. Stay away from caffeine, especially after one o'clock in the afternoon. Some of my colleagues argue, "I can drink a cup of coffee and go right to bed and fall asleep." The fact remains, though, that it will still rob you of your REM sleep, making your sleep nonrestorative. Because of this, you will feel down and drowsy the next day, all day, and need more caffeine, which will again interfere with your sleep. This vicious cycle will continue through your career and lead to suboptimal leadership and a truncated life. Please taper off caffeine slowly over three to four weeks to avoid withdrawal symptoms. Switch to decaf coffee if you must drink it.

- **Do not take over-the-counter sleeping pills without consulting your doctor.** An ideal sleeping pill is one that gives you six to eight hours of sleep with a normal percentage of deep sleep without causing daytime grogginess. It is also important that any sleeping pill you choose does not lose effectiveness with time and does not lead to dependence. Your physician can help you decide the right medication at the right dosage. Remember, you should not take a sleeping pill without knowing the cause of your insomnia. And when you do take a sleeping pill, take it at the lowest possible dosage for the shortest duration.

- **If you are interested in herbal supplements,** please read about valerian root, chamomile tea, and melatonin. You can visit the website of the National Center for Complementary and Alternative Medicine (NCCAM)[12] at http://nccam.nih.gov for more information. Chamomile is commonly used as a bedtime tea, but scientific evidence of its effectiveness for insomnia is lacking. The herb kava has been used for insomnia, but there is no evidence of its efficacy. The Food and Drug Administration (FDA) has issued a warning that kava supplements have been linked to a risk of severe liver damage. Valerian is one of the most popular herbal therapies for insomnia. Several studies suggest that valerian can improve the quality of sleep and slightly reduce the time it takes to fall asleep. However, not all the evidence is positive. One systematic review of the research concluded that, although valerian is commonly used as a sleep aid, the scientific evidence does not support its efficacy for insomnia. Researchers have concluded that valerian appears to be safe at recommended doses for short-term use. Some sleep-formula products combine valerian with other herbs, such as hops.

---

12 NCCAM is the federal government's lead agency for scientific research on the diverse medical and health-care systems, practices, and products that are not generally considered part of conventional medicine.

lavender, lemon balm, and skullcap. Although many of these other herbs have sedative properties, there is no reliable evidence that they improve insomnia or that combination products are more effective than valerian alone. Remember that the FDA has not tested the efficacy and safety of these supplements. Discuss these with your doctor.

- **Smell the candles**. Recognize that aromatherapy, using essential oils from herbs such as lavender or chamomile, is a popular sleep aid. Preliminary research suggests some sleep-inducing effects, but more studies are needed.
- **Listen to the music.** Listening to relaxing music of your choice at bedtime can help too. YouTube has a ten-minute music video by Dr. Jeffrey Thompson with more than eight million hits and great reviews from people suffering from insomnia. (You can check it out by searching "Jeffrey Thompson" on www.youtube.com.)

- **Learn progressive muscle relaxation.**

This is especially important if anxiety is contributing to your insomnia, because muscle relaxation is incompatible with anxiety. The technique is simple: Lie flat on your back in bed with your arms resting at your sides. Slowly breathe in and out. One by one, tighten and then completely and pleasantly relax each muscle, starting with the scalp muscle and moving down to the face muscles, neck, shoulder, chest, arms, abdomen, back, legs, and all the way to the toe muscles. You can repeat this process several times until you achieve complete relaxation. The goal is to achieve a sense of complete weightlessness through total physical and mental relaxation, and thereby eliminate anxiety. You can also try total relaxation, demonstrated in a ten-minute video on YouTube posted by Nancy Parker (coolkarmavideo is her YouTube user name).

- **Learn Mindfulness Meditation**

You can learn the technique on www.shambhalasun.com. You can also search for instructional videos on www.youtube.com that teach to meditation techniques. A six-minute guided instructional video by Jim Malloy (jmalloy108) is extremely helpful.

"Mindfulness practice is simple and completely feasible. Just by sitting and doing nothing, we are doing a tremendous amount."

In mindfulness, or shamatha, meditation, we are trying to achieve a mind that is stable and calm. What we begin to discover is that this calmness or harmony is a natural aspect of the mind. Through mindfulness practice we are just developing and strengthening it, and eventually we are able to remain peacefully in our mind without struggling. Our mind naturally feels content. Here are a few tips to help you get started.

- Create a favorable environment. It is good if the place where you meditate, even if it's only a small space in your apartment, has a feeling of sacredness.

  Begin with baby steps. I encourage people to meditate frequently but for short periods of time—ten, fifteen, or twenty minutes. If you force it too much, the practice can take on too much of a personality, and training the mind should be very, very simple.
- Create a sense of discipline. When we sit down, we can remind ourselves: "I'm here to work on my mind. I'm here to train my mind." It's OK to say that to yourself when you sit down, literally. We need that kind of inspiration as we begin to practice.

- Maintain an erect posture. The Buddhist approach is that the mind and body are connected. The energy flows better when the body is erect, and when it's bent, the flow is changed and that directly affects your thought process. People who need to use a chair for meditation should sit upright with their feet touching the ground. Those using a meditation cushion such as a zafu or gomden should find a comfortable position with legs crossed and hands resting palm-down on your thighs. The hips are neither rotated forward too much, nor tilted back so you start slouching. You should have a feeling of stability and strength.
- Maintain a soft downward gaze. For strict mindfulness practice, the gaze should be downward focusing a couple of inches in front of your nose. The eyes are open but not staring; your gaze is soft. We are trying to reduce sensory input as much as we can.

- Focus on your breathing. When we do shamatha practice, we become more and more familiar with our mind, and in particular we learn to recognize the movement of the mind, which we experience as thoughts. We do this by using an object of meditation to provide a contrast or counterpoint to what's happening in our mind. As soon as we go off and start thinking about something, awareness of the object of meditation will bring us back. We could put a rock in front of us and use it to focus our mind, but using the breath as the object of meditation is particularly helpful because it relaxes us. As you start the practice, you have a sense of your body and a sense of where you are, and then you begin to notice the breathing. The whole feeling of the breath is very important. The breath should not be forced, obviously; you are breathing naturally. The breath is going in and out, in and out. With each breath you become relaxed.

- Ignore your thoughts. No matter what kind of thought comes up, you should say to yourself, "That may be a really important issue in my life, but right now is not the time to think about it. Now I'm practicing meditation." It gets down to how honest we are, how true we can be to ourselves, during each session. Everyone gets lost in thought sometimes. You might think, "I can't believe I got so absorbed in something like that," but try not to make it too personal. Just try to be as unbiased as possible. The mind will be wild and we have to recognize that. We can't push ourselves. We notice that we have been lost in thought, we mentally label it "thinking"—gently and without judgment—and we come back to the breath. When we have a thought—no matter how wild or bizarre it may be—we just let it go and come back to the breath, come back to the situation here.

What we are talking about is very practical. Mindfulness practice is simple and completely feasible. And because we are working with the mind that experiences life directly, just by sitting and doing nothing, we are doing a tremendous amount.

By Sakyong Jamgon Mipham Rinpoche, the great nineteenth-century Buddhist teacher. Published in the January 2000 issue of the *Shambhala Sun.*

Consult your doctor if you have sleep apnea based on the STOP questionnaire, insomnia that persists beyond a week, have fallen asleep driving or come close to it, have fallen asleep during meetings, or felt sleepy and tired in the afternoon or evening.

We have a built-in reluctance to seek help when it comes to our own health. We are used to being in charge. We like to call the shots. We will tough it out. We will suffer. We will do everything but seek help from a doctor. "No one tells me what to do," we say.

Please overcome that inhibition and see a doctor to design a plan of action; then stick to it. Your life, your family, and your friends need you to be maximally alert all day long.

- **Conquer Procrastination**

At some point this common ailment of procrastination has inflicted us. We have known the deadline for several weeks, but we find reasons not to work on that project until the last night, and then we pull an all-nighter and give an acceptable final product, but one that is far from being the best our creative mind can provide.

"I work best under pressure." We all have heard this, and it is true. But the problem is that when there is time pressure, we have adrenaline overflow, which increases our output but kills our creativity. We can analyze piles of data rapidly, discuss each point thoroughly, and put together the final presentation quickly, but the creativity is conspicuously absent. The big-picture vision is not there. The out-of-the-box thinking is still at home on our pillow.

Procrastination actually increases the energy required to complete a project. If project A requires *x* amount of intellectual energy, *y* amount of physical energy, and *z* amount of emotional energy, then, with procrastination, the same project will require the same amount of intellectual and physical energy, but a much larger amount of emotional energy because this incomplete, unpleasant task continually haunts your subconscious.

The energy required to complete **project A** = $x + y + z$. With procrastination, the energy required to complete **project A** = $x + y + z^t$, where t is time taken to finish the project. Why does this happen? It is the result of a psychological defense mechanism that compels us to avoid tasks that are unpleasant, difficult, emotionally demanding, or anxiety provoking. Maybe deep down we fear we will fail in providing a perfect presentation Maybe we are afraid of failure and subsequent humiliation.

Conquering procrastination is difficult, but here are a few suggestions to help you get started:

- Replace negative emotions with enthusiasm by using faith, peer support, and incessant activity, both physical and intellectual.
- Set pseudo-deadlines. I have found this immensely helpful when dealing with an unpleasant project. Tell yourself and your teammates that the deadline is a week before the actual deadline.
- Start small. A series of small steps will generate confidence and motivate you to finish the big project.

- Use "front loaders" first. If it is a team project, assign "front loaders" the task of researching and writing the preliminary draft, while assigning the polishing of the final product to the "back loaders." This way, at least the front loaders will present the project well rested.

A Fun Fact

Did you know that the second week of March is National Procrastination Week? Well, actually, it's the first week of March, but it is celebrated in the second week after a lot of procrastination. *Happy front loading!*

- **Manage Time Well to Get More REM**

If you want to lead with excellence, then you know you must master time management. How are your time-management skills these days? Are you one of those rare people who seem to have it all together and get everything accomplished on their to-do list, and still have time left over at the end of the day? Following are some tips to help you find more time:

- Recognize that your time is exactly that—your time. If you are like most people, there are those in your life who have no respect for your time. Those include the people who are always asking you to do something for them. Until you learn how to just say no, they will continue to rob you of your time. Hence, learn and then practice saying no. (*A "no" uttered from the deepest conviction is better than a "yes" merely uttered to please, or worse, to avoid trouble. —Gandhi*) Please yourself first, because you deserve it. Once you stop trying to please everyone else, you will start freeing up time in your own schedule.
- Look for ways you can combine tasks to save time. Simple things like reading the newspaper while riding the train to work, or taping your favorite television shows (and then fast-forwarding through the commercials) will give you more time. Be creative; see how many ways you can save time next week.
- If you are working on a project on a computer, resist the urge to keep checking your e-mail. Those e-mail distractions will keep you from getting your project completed on time.

- Turn off the television for at least an hour in the evening. Do not let the television networks control your nightly schedule. Be the true master of the remote control.

- **Discipline Results in Deep Sleep**

Inadequate sleep hygiene is a major contributor to sleep disturbance and deprivation. Daytime sleepiness and difficulty falling asleep at night are solid indicators of poor sleep hygiene.

Sleep hygiene is just a matter of following simple and sensible guidelines. The result will help ensure more restful, restorative sleep, and promote greater daytime productivity and attentiveness.

- **Learn the Benefits of a Power Nap**

Winston Churchill said, "A nap in the afternoon gives you two days in one." While talking to Dan Rather of CBS News in 1993, Bill Clinton said, "If I can take a nap—even fifteen or twenty minutes—in the middle of the day, it is really invigorating to me. On the days when I'm a little short of sleep, I try to work it out so that I can sneak off and just lie down for fifteen minutes, a half hour, and it really makes all the difference in the world."

Because of our circadian rhythm, our alertness and, hence, our performance dips in the afternoon. This nadir is deeper when we are sleep deprived and when we are traveling across multiple time zones. If we can fight this drowsiness with a strategically placed power nap, then we can maximize executive function and avoid fatal mistakes. (Most fatal vehicular accidents occur in the midafternoon and after midnight.)

Studies prove that a fifteen-minute power nap provides benefits lasting up to 150 minutes, including:

- Improved alertness, both subjectively and objectively
- Reduced fatigue and improved vigor
- Enhanced creativity and problem solving

- Improved perception[13]
- Facilitated learning
- Improved declarative and procedural memory
- Positive mood and emotions, clearer communication, humor and optimism, and situational awareness

If a fifteen-minute nap gives you 150 minutes of improved executive function, how can you resist such an investment?

- **Overcome the Cultural Barrier to Power Napping**

The biggest obstacle to the practice of power napping is the stigma it carries in our frenzied corporate culture, which looks at napping as a sign of weakness, not wisdom. How do you take a power nap then? As with most changes, this one also begins in your mind. Review the reasons for power naps and the benefits they offer. Analyze the data and make a rational decision. Next, share your plan to invest in power naps with people around you, starting with your spouse, your secretary, your closest colleague, and so on.

---

[13] Using a functional MRI, a study by Dr. Sara Mednik showed that a nap prevents perception fatigue.

As appropriate, educate your staff and colleagues about the performance benefits of power naps. Inform them that napping is a sign of wisdom, not weakness. This will help you overcome that cultural barrier and stigma associated with daytime napping. Then show the confidence of a leader and just do it.[14] It is not that difficult; and it is worth the trouble and time.

- **Learn to Take PREM (Patel's Relaxed Eye Muscles) Nap**

But how do you take this power nap? Relax. It's easy. You don't have to do anything hard. Of course, there is a definite learning curve, but you will get better as you take these power naps on a regular basis.

In research studies, participants were asked to take naps in a quiet, dark, and comfortable environment. You may not have such an environment at work, but with practice, you can still take a very invigorating and rewarding nap. Legend has it that a ferocious Mughal warrior, Aurangzeb, took naps while still sitting on his horse in the middle of the battlefield.

---

[14] If you are not in the corner office yet, you can use your lunch break to take a power nap!

The following tips will help you rejuvenate your day with a fifteen-minute power nap:

- Proudly let your staff know that you will be taking a fifteen-minute nap. "Doctor's orders," you may add.
- Set your phone alarm, preferably on vibrate, to go off in fifteen minutes. An Australian study has shown that napping for less than ten minutes is suboptimal. More than twenty minutes can be counterproductive because of post-nap grogginess.
- Turn on relaxing music. You can try noise-canceling headphones. Bose are the best.
- Put on an eyeshade. I find my Notre Dame cap very useful, especially when taking a nap in a public place; I just pull it down over my eyes, and I am off to the land of dreams.
- Stretch out on a couch or recline in a chair. Turn the chair away from people and toward the window or wall. A study from China showed greater benefit with stretching on the couch, as opposed to sitting.
- Close your eyes, shut off your mind, and relax.
- Wake up with a smile and vigor when the alarm goes off.

- Before the nap, read a couple of lines from the Bible or another religious book. You can store them on your smartphone and read them before setting up the fifteen-minute alarm. Unfortunately, REM sleep, the sleep stage with vivid dreams, predominantly produces negative emotions such as fear, anxiety, guilt, and anger. This reading will help replace them with joy, optimism, love, and faith.
- Begin your nap with five to ten slow, deep, regular breaths. Control of breathing is control of life. Breathing, unlike heart rate, blood pressure, temperature, and gastrointestinal motility/secretions, is the only vital function that we can easily control, and it is a time-tested tool used for centuries to achieve relaxation.
- Progressive muscle relaxation is incompatible with somatic anxiety. So, by focusing on respiration and relaxation, we are getting rid of anxiety, both from our conscious and our subconscious. As you breathe in and out, relax the muscles of your eyeballs and then continue to relax all the other muscles from head to toe and drift down into a state of pleasant relaxation. And when the alarm goes off, wake up with tremendous positive energy. I call this my PREM nap!

Here is how PREM nap compares to conventional nap.

Conventional Nap:	**PREM Nap:**
Slower cooling off	Rapid cooling off
Negative emotions	Positive emotions
Irregular respirations	Regular respirations
Incomplete muscle relaxation	Complete muscle relaxation
Untapped spiritual energy	Taps into spiritual energy

- **Tackle Tough Problems after a PREM Nap**

As we saw earlier, a nap containing REM sleep improves creative problem solving by a whopping 40 percent.

Remember that REM sleep has an active brain in a paralyzed body. Mother Nature made it so we do not act out our dreams. Also, studies have shown that REM sleep has a tremendous amount of random, bizarre, and seemingly unrelated activity, which our brain is trying to connect to make some sense of. Some researchers believe this is why a REM nap is able to boost creative problem solving; it links these random and totally unrelated activities together. This is the wildest and craziest form of thinking outside the box. Studies have shown that REM sleep plays a pivotal role in memory consolidation too.

- **Practice Open-eye Nap**

Once you have mastered the PREM nap, the next big challenge is to learn to take a PREM nap with open eyes[15] in a public place! Imagine you are listening to a long, dull PowerPoint presentation that is not going to help your cause, but you cannot get up and leave. Or you are done giving your speech, and as a courtesy to the other speakers, you remain until the entire function is over. You have a ton of things to do as soon as the presentation is done. Can you nap for three to four minutes at a time with your eyes open, and use these minutes to recharge your executive engine? Why not? Fish sleep with their eyes open. A giraffe sleeps while standing. You can do that too.

The open-eye nap does become easier after you have tried the PREM nap for a month or two, but for now, get started using the following techniques:

---

[15] Vice President Joe Biden was caught napping during a budget speech by President Obama. He should have used the open-eye nap!

- Sit in a comfortable position. Sitting upright is fine. If the situation permits, you can slide down in the chair too; just make sure the chair does not slide away.
- Pleasantly focus your eyes on the screen or toward the podium. Remember, when we sleep, our ears are open, and we still sleep well. Here, both your eyes and ears are open. With practice, you can successfully shut off your mind and relax completely.
- Take slow, deep breaths and relax from head to toe. Do not worry. You will not fall down. The tone of spinal muscles will hold you in the chair.

What if someone asks you a direct question? Do not worry. You will be able to wake up and respond, just as a sleeping mother can ignore everything else, but hears and responds to her child's crying in the next room. Before responding, you can say, "I'm sorry, I was still thinking about the excellent point you made earlier. Can you repeat your question, please?" You can also ask a trusted neighbor or a team member to come to your rescue should there be a question or a comment directed at you. Just say, "Please tap my knee or shoulder if there is a question or comment I should respond to. I might be absorbed in some other thoughts."

Happy napping!

In this section, we learned about the importance of getting sound sleep of sufficient duration, and following sleep-hygiene instructions that can help us achieve quality sleep. In the next section, we will learn about the unique problems faced by females and how you can get sound sleep during those specific situations. So let's get started.

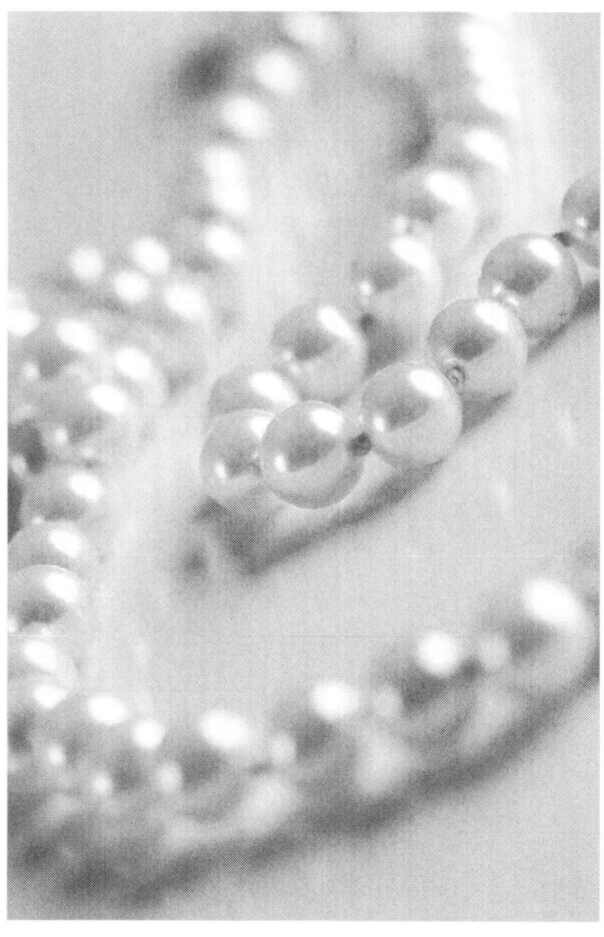

Section III
"It's a Female Thing. You Wouldn't Understand."

- Sleep Soundly Despite PMS and Menstruation
- Sleep Well When Sleeping for Two
- Help Baby Sleep through the Night
- Sleep Well during Menopause and Beyond
- Sleep Better Despite Fibromyalgia

- **Sleep Soundly Despite PMS and Menstruation**

According to the National Sleep Foundation's Women and Sleep poll, half of menstruating women complain of disrupted sleep for three days during each menstrual cycle. For female leaders suffering from premenstrual syndrome, sleep disruption and the resultant drop in daytime alertness are even worse. Also, the hormone progesterone, which peaks during the second half of the menstrual cycle, exacerbates fatigue and excessive daytime sleepiness. These recurring challenges can take a toll on leadership and the life of our female leaders.

The following pearls can help. Remember that if you master these interventions, you get recurring return on your investment month after month throughout your life:

- Follow sleep hygiene with a fervor. Mother Nature is not helping you, so you will have to help yourself.
- Remember that exercise will help fight PMS symptoms and improve your REM sleep.
- Gradually taper off caffeine completely. Besides disrupting your deep sleep, caffeine contributes to premenstrual bloating.
- Drink more during the daytime. Drink plenty of fluids all day, but stop drinking in the evening to avoid nocturnal urination.

- Avoid the it-is-just-PMS attitude. Take your PMS seriously, and consult your physician to reduce PMS symptoms of bloating, breast tenderness, back pain, cramping, irritability, nervousness, and grumpiness.
- Schedule lightly. You may argue that this is not always possible, but with proper planning, you might be able to achieve this. Try to squeeze in a PREM nap in your busy schedule if you can.
- Do not let pride prevent you from seeking support. You know you are fighting Mother Nature, but no one else does because you cannot share this with your male colleagues. This should not prevent you from seeking support from your female colleagues and, for sure, your family members.
- Learn mindfulness meditation. It will help you deal with untoward emotions and will also treat that feeling of powerlessness.

- **Sleep Well When Sleeping for Two**

Pregnancy can severely affect the quality and quantity of your executive output because of poor sleep resulting from hormonal and other physiological changes your body goes through during pregnancy. According to the National Sleep Foundation's 1998 Women and Sleep poll, 78 percent of women reported more disturbed sleep during pregnancy than at other times. Following are the common problems responsible for disturbed sleep during pregnancy:

1. **Insomnia.** Women may report difficulty falling asleep, staying asleep, waking up too early, or waking up tired. Stress or anxiety about labor, delivery, and motherhood may result in significant sleep loss. The discomforts of pregnancy, such as nausea, back pain, and fetal movements, may also disturb sleep.
2. **Restless leg syndrome (RLS).** Symptoms of restless leg syndrome include unpleasant feelings in the legs, sometimes described as creepy, tingly, or achy. These feelings are worse at night or in the hours before bedtime. Movement or stretching temporarily relieves them. In a study of more than six hundred pregnant women, 26 percent reported symptoms of RLS.

3. **Sleep apnea.** Hormonal changes relax your upper airway muscles, which may result in snoring and sleep apnea (repeated cessation of respirations lasting for ten or more seconds and robbing you of your deep sleep, causing severe daytime sleepiness and fatigue). Untreated, sleep apnea also increases the risk of gestational hypertension, preeclampsia, and low birth weight. Answer the following questions; if you reply yes to two or more, you are at high risk for obstructive sleep apnea and should talk to your doctor. A simple home sleep test can diagnose this serious disease. There is a safe, easy, and very effective treatment called continuous positive airway pressure (CPAP). CPAP hooks to a nasal mask or cannula, which acts as a pneumatic splint that keeps the airway open, thus eliminating snoring, sleep apnea, sleep disruption, and the apnea-related complications.

S—Do you **snore** loudly?

T—Do you often feel **tired**, fatigued, or sleepy during the daytime?

O—Has anyone **observed** you stop breathing during sleep?

P—Do you have or are you being treated for high blood **pressure**?

4. **Nocturnal gastroesophageal reflux (nighttime GERD).** Also known as heartburn, GERD is considered a normal part of pregnancy. However, nighttime symptoms of GERD can damage the esophagus and disrupt sleep during pregnancy. One study found that 30–50 percent of pregnant women experience GERD almost constantly during pregnancy.
5. **Frequent nighttime urination.** The frequent need to urinate at night is a common feature of pregnancy and can result in loss of sleep.
6. **Rising progesterone levels.** These exacerbate fatigue, tiredness, and excessive daytime sleepiness, especially in the first trimester.

Sleeping well throughout your pregnancy can be challenging. Use these pearls throughout your pregnancy to minimize loss of sleep:

- Plan, schedule, and prioritize sleep. Follow sleep hygiene with twice the fervor and fanaticism, as you are indeed sleeping for two.
- Avoid caffeine completely because it will compound the problem of insufficient deep sleep. Being a diuretic, caffeine will also increase your frequency of urination.

- After checking with your physician, exercise for at least thirty minutes per day.
- Sleep on your left side to improve the flow of blood and nutrients to your fetus and your uterus and kidneys. Keep your knees and hips bent. Place pillows between your knees, under your abdomen, and behind your back; this may take pressure off your lower back. Try to avoid lying on your back for extended periods of time. You may try special pregnancy pillows, which can help you be comfortable during sleep.
- Drink lots of fluids during the day, especially water, but cut down on the amount you drink in the hours before bedtime.
- If you can't get to sleep for twenty minutes, don't lie in bed and force yourself to sleep. Get out of the bedroom and read a relaxing book, knit or crochet something for your baby, write in a journal, or take a warm bath.
- Learn progressive muscle relaxation. This will help your insomnia, and it will come in handy during delivery.
- Avoid looking at bright light at night. A night-light in the bathroom will be less stimulating, allowing you to return to sleep more quickly.

- On workdays, take a PREM power nap in the early afternoon. On weekends, you can take a longer nap in the afternoon to pay up your sleep debt. If you have difficulty falling asleep at night, then nap earlier in the day or curtail the duration of the nap.
- To avoid heartburn, do not eat large amounts of spicy, acidic, or fried foods. Also, eat frequent small meals throughout the day.
- Recognize that snoring is very common during pregnancy, but if you have pauses in your breathing associated with your snoring, you should be screened for sleep apnea.
- If you develop RLS, seek medical attention. Your doctor will check you for iron or folate deficiency.
- Keep your legs elevated at work and at home as much as you can. This can prevent leg swelling and may help your RLS. Leg-stretching exercises can help RLS too.

God bless you both!

Help Baby Sleep through the Night

If you haven't had a good night's sleep since your baby was born, you're not alone. Sleepless nights are a rite of passage for most new parents—but don't despair. You can help your baby sleep all night. Honestly! Use these simple tips as suggested by the Mayo Clinic to help your baby sleep through the night.

o Learn about Baby's Developing Rhythm

Newborns sleep sixteen or more hours a day, but often in stretches of just a few hours at a time. Although the pattern might be erratic at first, a more consistent sleep schedule will emerge as your baby matures and can go longer between feedings.

By age three months, many babies sleep at least five hours at a time. By age six months, nighttime stretches of nine to twelve hours are possible.

- **Encourage Good Sleep Habits**

For the first few months, middle-of-the-night feedings are sure to disrupt sleep for parents and babies alike—but it's never too soon to help your baby become a good sleeper. Consider using these pearls:

- Encourage activity during the day. When your baby is awake, engage him or her by talking, singing, and playing. Stimulation during the day can help promote better sleep at night.
- Follow a consistent bedtime routine. Try relaxing favorites such as bathing, cuddling, singing, playing quiet music, or reading. Soon your baby will associate these activities with sleep.
- Put your baby to bed drowsy but awake. This will help your baby associate bed with the process of falling asleep. Remember to place your baby to sleep on his or her back, and clear the crib or bassinet of blankets and other soft items.
- Give your baby time to settle down. Your baby might fuss or cry before finding a comfortable position and falling asleep. If the crying doesn't stop, speak to your baby calmly and stroke his or her back. Your reassuring presence might be all your baby needs to fall asleep.

- Consider a pacifier. If your baby has trouble settling down, a pacifier might do the trick. In fact, research suggests that using a pacifier during sleep helps reduce the risk of sudden infant death syndrome (SIDS).
- Expect frequent stirring at night. Babies often wriggle, squirm, and twitch in their sleep. They can be noisy too. Unless you suspect that your baby is hungry or uncomfortable, it's OK to wait a few minutes to see if he or she falls back asleep.
- Keep nighttime care low-key. When your baby needs care or feeding during the night, use dim lights, a soft voice, and calm movements. This will tell your baby that it's time to sleep—not play.
- Don't "bed share" during sleep. This can make it harder for your baby to fall asleep on his or her own. Bed sharing might also increase your baby's risk of SIDS. If you'd like to keep your baby close, consider placing your baby's bed in your bedroom.
- Respect your baby's preferences. If your baby is a night owl or an early bird, you might want to adjust routines and schedules based on these natural patterns.

- **Keep It in Perspective**

Getting your baby to sleep through the night is a worthy goal, but it's not a measure of your parenting skills. Take time to understand your baby's habits and ways of communicating so that you can help him or her become a better sleeper. If you continue to have concerns, consult your baby's doctor for additional suggestions.

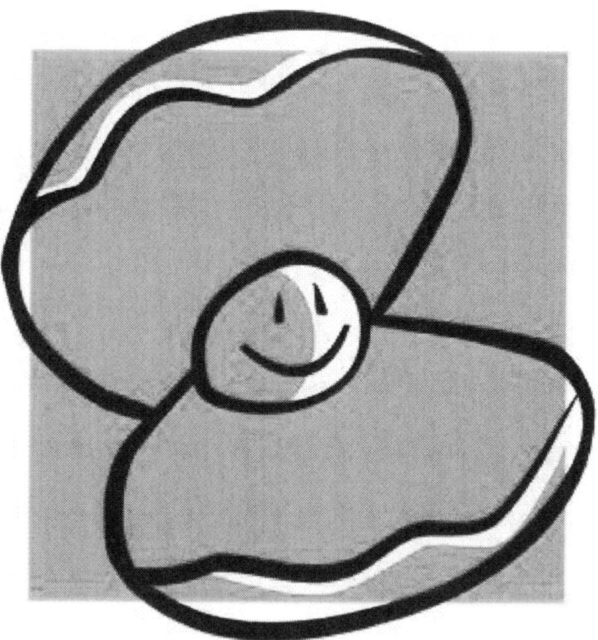

Sleep Well during Menopause and Beyond

During the transition phase leading to menopause over several years, a woman's ovaries gradually decrease production of estrogen and progesterone. A woman reaches menopause one year after menstrual periods have stopped, usually around the age of fifty. Menopause is a time of major hormonal, physical, and psychological change. Natural changes in sleep also occur, characterized by longer time to sleep onset, frequent awakenings, decreased amount of deep sleep, and poor sleep architecture. From perimenopause to postmenopause, women report hot flashes, mood disorders, insomnia, and sleep-disordered breathing. Sleep problems are often accompanied by depression and anxiety, which make insomnia worse. This is the reason postmenopausal women are less satisfied with their sleep and why as many as 61 percent report insomnia symptoms. Snoring and sleep apnea have also been found to be more common and more severe in postmenopausal women because their upper airway dilator muscles become flabby with aging.

Changing and decreasing levels of estrogen cause many menopausal symptoms, including hot flashes, which are unexpected feelings of heat all over the body, accompanied by sweating. They usually begin around the face and spread to the chest, affecting 75–85 percent of women around menopause. On average, hot flashes last three minutes and lead to less sleep efficiency. Most women experience these for one year, but about 25 percent have hot flashes for five years. Hot flashes interrupt sleep and reduce the amount of deep sleep, leading to suboptimal alertness and suboptimal life the following day.

Talk to your doctor about estrogen (estrogen replacement therapy, or ERT) or estrogen and progesterone (hormone replacement therapy, or HRT), nutritional products, and medications such as calcium supplements, vitamin D, and bisphosphonates for the prevention or treatment of osteoporosis (thinning and weakening of the bones). Also discuss estrogen creams and rings for vaginal dryness, as well as alternative treatment for menopausal symptoms, such as soy products (tofu, soybeans, and soy milk), which contain phytoestrogen, a plant hormone similar to estrogen. Soy products may lessen hot flashes. Phytoestrogens are also available in over-the-counter nutritional supplements (ginseng, extract of red clover, and black cohosh). The FDA does not regulate these supplements. Their proper doses, safety, and long-term effects and risks are not yet known.

Typically, a leader's career spans five to six decades. And toward the later part of your career, because of your vast experience, a lifelong network of experts, and the wisdom that comes only with age, you are worth more than you ever were. This makes it imperative that you take good care of your sleep and your health so you can continue to contribute to the welfare of the human race; in other words, take your menopausal symptoms seriously and seek professional help.

Here are a few pearls to help you sleep well:

- Continue to follow sleep hygiene and insomnia instructions.
- Avoid foods that are spicy or acidic because these may trigger hot flashes. Try foods rich in soy because they might minimize hot flashes.
- Avoid nicotine, caffeine, and alcohol, especially before bedtime. These will make your hot flashes worse.
- Dress in lightweight clothes to improve sleep efficiency. Avoid heavy, insulating blankets, and consider using a fan or air conditioner to cool the air and increase circulation. If your spouse is shivering, place a small portable heater next to his side of the bed. Manufacturers of the Sleep Number bed have come out with a mattress with separate temperature controls for you and your spouse.
- Reduce stress and worry as much as possible. Try relaxation techniques, massage, and exercise. Talk to a behavioral health professional if you are depressed, anxious, or having problems.
- Try consolidating your sleep by going to bed thirty minutes later than your usual bedtime. As we age, we spend more time in bed, but sleep less.

Sleep Better Despite Fibromyalgia

Fibromyalgia is a chronic, debilitating, frustrating syndrome characterized by long-term, body-wide pain and tenderness in the joints, muscles, tendons, and other soft tissues. These aches and pains lead to sleep onset and sleep maintenance difficulties, which in turn exacerbate the aches and pains perpetuating the vicious cycle. A unique phenomenon we see during the sleep study of these patients is the frequent intrusion of alpha waves (fast brain waves usually seen during wakefulness) into the delta waves (Slow and synchronous brain waves characteristic of deep sleep.) This makes the sleep nonrestorative leading to fatigue, tiredness, excessive sleepiness, and achiness the next day. Here are my pearls for the patients suffering from this challenging disorder.

- Follow the sleep hygiene instructions religiously. Others in your family do not suffer from fibromyalgia, but you unfortunately do. You have to follow good habits on a daily basis.
- Caffeine will make those frequent arousals and awakenings worse. Taper it off completely.
- Learn progressive muscle relaxation and the mindfulness meditation, both discussed earlier in this book.

- See a sleep physician to discuss if a sleeping pill is a good option. The sleep physician will help you choose the best sedating medication with fewest side effects. The sleep physician will also discuss sleep hygiene instructions, sleep education, sleep restriction, stimulus control, and guided imagery as applicable to your particular situation. You can learn more about these techniques at the Mayo Clinic website, www.mayoclinic.com/health/insomnia-treatment/SL00013. These techniques have been shown to be more effective than sleeping pills in promoting sound sleep in patients suffering from insomnia. It does take effort and discipline to learn and implement these techniques, but it is worth the reward.
- Talk to a behavior therapist.

Cognitive-behavioral therapy is an important part of treatment. This therapy helps you learn how to:

- Deal with negative thoughts
- Keep a diary of pain and symptoms
- Recognize what makes your symptoms worse
- Seek out enjoyable activities
- Set limits

- Discuss with your primary physician about a referral to a rheumatologist, a pain specialist, or an acupuncturist as appropriate.
- Talk to a physical therapist and design an exercise program that suits your individual case. Exercise training can include aerobics such as stepping and walking; strengthening exercises such as lifting weights or using resistance machines; and stretching for flexibility. Although exercise is part of the overall management of fibromyalgia, this review examined the effects of exercise when used separately or combined with other strategies such as education programs, biofeedback and medications.

In the studies, aerobic exercises were done for at least twenty minutes once a day (or twice for at least ten minutes), two or three days a week. Strength training was done two or three times a week and with at least eight to twelve repetitions per exercise. The exercise programs lasted between two and a half to twenty-four weeks.

- Learn the benefits of aerobic exercise training. Studies have shown that the exercise training may:
    1. Improve overall wellbeing by 7 points on a scale of 0 to 100.

2. Improve ability to perform aerobic exercise, by using 2.8 ml/kg/minute more oxygen when walking on a treadmill.
3. Increase the amount of pressure that can be applied to a tender point by 0.23 kg/cm^2 before the onset of pain.
4. Reduce pain by 1.3 on a scale of 0 to 10.

- Learn the benefits of strength training. When compared to no exercise, strength training may:
    1. Reduce pain by 49 fewer points on a scale of 0 to 100.
    2. Improve overall wellbeing by 41 points on a scale of 0 to 100.
    3. Lead to 2 fewer active tender points on a scale of 0 to 18.

In this section, we learned about the unique problems faced by females and how to tackle those problems to get a sufficient amount of deep sleep. In the next section, we will learn about sleep deprivation; its causes, deleterious effects, and the countermeasures you can use. So let us get started.

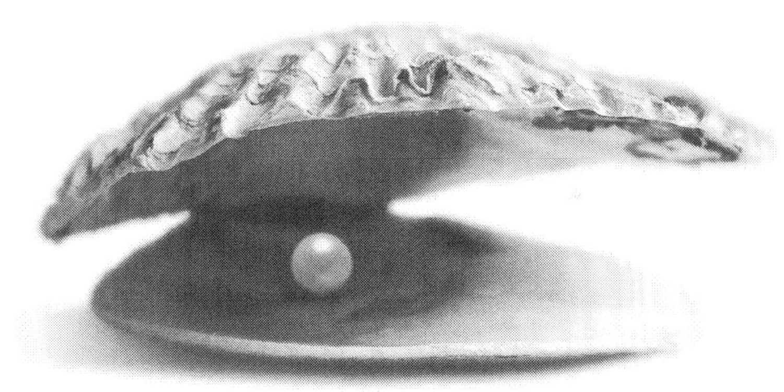

Section IV

Insufficient Sleep, Incomplete Life

- Beware of Poor Sleep's Side Effects
- Know Your Sleep Debt
- Regain Your Family Life
- Learn from Politician's Mistakes
- Get Treated for Obstructive Sleep Apnea
- Eliminate Bad Sleep Habits
- Eliminate Insomnia of Interpersonal Conflict
- Sleep Soundly Even during Excitement
- Eliminate Anxiety about Falling Sleep

Sleep deprivation is defined as a sufficient lack of restorative sleep over a cumulative period so as to cause physical or psychiatric symptoms and affect routine performances of tasks. If your brain needs eight hours of sleep and it gets seven and a half, it suffers from quantitative sleep deprivation and resulting ill effects on leadership. Interestingly, if your brain needs eight hours of sleep and gets eight hours of poor-quality sleep (less REM sleep percentage than normal) because of poor sleep hygiene, then it suffers from qualitative sleep deprivation. Most of our female colleagues suffer from both qualitative and quantitative sleep deprivation. They keep collecting sleep debt, which, unfortunately, is cumulative and cannot be paid off in one lump sum by sleeping in over the weekend.

o Beware of Poor Sleep's Side Effects

In general, poor sleep results in:

1. Lapsing, cognitive slowing,[16] memory impairment, and reduced vigilance[17]
2. Change in mood and motivation, failure to complete routines, slower responses, physical exertion, and bickering
3. Increased reaction time and decreased vigilance and attention
4. Impaired working memory, verbal fluency,[18] logical reasoning, decision making, and judgment
5. Decrements in innovative, flexible thinking, and strategic planning[19]
6. Increased perseveration (trying failed solutions repeatedly) and lack of flexibility[20]

---

[16] Slowed-down thought processes.

[17] Vitally important for pilots, surgeons, and executives in a board meeting.

[18] Our speech becomes incomprehensible at times.

[19] Effect has been shown after one night without sleep.

[20] Effect has been shown after one night of sleep loss, even on tests lasting less than ten minutes.

7. Inability to focus on greater good, and resultant indecisiveness when faced with an ethical dilemma
8. Inability to set ambitious goals
9. Diminished problem-solving abilities
10. Severely diminished ability to manage information
11. Reactive instead of proactive response
12. Diminished verbal fluency and communication skills
13. Emotional agnosia (inability to recognize and manage emotions)
14. Impaired mood, cognition, and psychomotor vigilance (makes you grumpy, foggy, and clumsy)

Because of the effect of sleep deprivation on the prefrontal cortex, sleep-deprived females lack the speed and creative resources to make quick, logical decisions and implement them well. These same studies indicate that a sleep-deprived person lacks the ability to consider multiple tasks simultaneously, which reduces the speed and efficiency of one's actions.

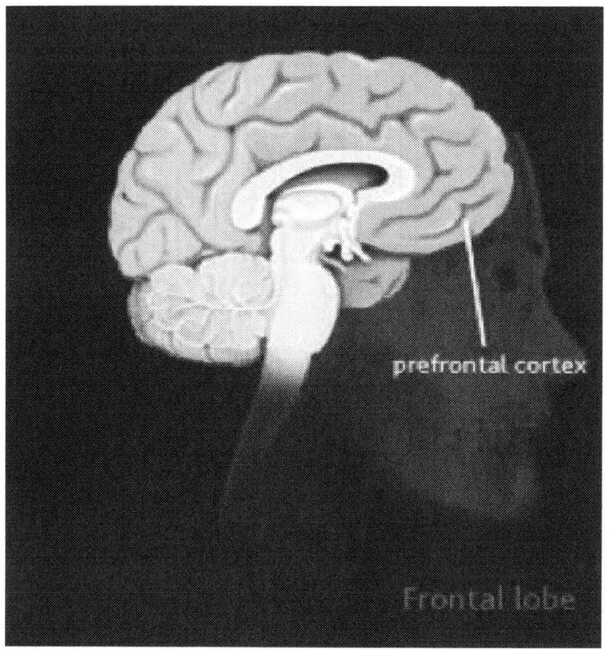

In studying the effects of sleep deprivation on the prefrontal cortex, researchers in the University of Iowa's Department of Neurology discovered that the prefrontal cortex of a sleep-deprived person functions much like a damaged prefrontal cortex. The only real difference is that sleep-deprived people have the ability to reset the prefrontal cortex's function simply by returning to a healthy amount of restorative sleep.

The bottom line is that sleep deprivation significantly reduces brain activity within the prefrontal cortex. This reduction of brain activity makes it just about impossible to make a correct decision, especially when the outcomes are uncertain. Think about that the next time you make a major career decision or long-term strategic decisions about your corporation in the presence of sleep deprivation.

- **Know Your Sleep Debt**

You can use the Epworth Sleepiness Scale (ESS) to determine the level of sleepiness you are experiencing because of cumulative sleep debt. ESS is a measure of chronic (long-term) sleepiness, while Patel's Alertness Sleepiness Scale (PASS) is a measure of sleepiness at a given moment. To find out your ESS, calculate your chance of dozing or sleeping in each situation described below.

Use this scale to choose the most appropriate number for each situation:

0 would never doze or sleep

1 slight chance of dozing or sleeping

2 moderate chance of dozing or sleeping

3 high chance of dozing or sleeping

Situation	**Chance of Dozing or Sleeping**
Sitting and reading	
Watching TV	
Sitting inactive in a public place	
Being a passenger in a motor vehicle for an hour or more	
Lying down in the afternoon	
Sitting and talking to someone	
Sitting quietly after lunch (no alcohol)	
Stopped for a few minutes in traffic while driving	
Total:	

Add up the numbers to determine your ESS score, which is a measure of sleep debt. A score of ten or more indicates suboptimal function as a result of sleep debt. If you score ten or more on this test, you should consider whether you are obtaining adequate sleep, need to improve your sleep hygiene, and/or see a sleep specialist. You should discuss these issues with your personal physician.

o Regain Your Family Life

Because it adversely affects every aspect of your life: professional, family, and personal. In fact, it affects your personal and family life even more than your professional life. When you are sleep deprived, you still have to do what you are paid to do, though it might be of suboptimal quality. There are enough layers of safety and support to ensure your work meets minimum safety and quality standards. But when you come home tired and sleep deprived, there is no such pressure to perform, no support system to help you, and no minimum standards you must reach. So you may skip your son's basketball game, cancel your customary walk with your husband, or fail to enjoy quality time at the dinner table.

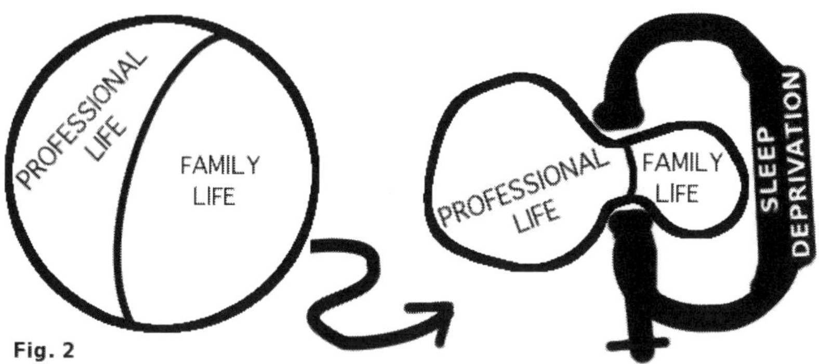

Sleep deprivation shrinks a leader's professional life and to a much greater extent, family life.

- **Learn from Politicians' Mistakes**

To get a glimpse of how sleep deprivation affects the human personality, think back to the 2008 US presidential campaign. Politicians from throughout the United States were on the trail, making speeches, kissing babies, and fending off negative ads designed to derail their campaigns. From early morning to late at night, these presidential candidates were giving it their all, with their lives under a microscope, and microphones, television cameras, and inquisitive reporters monitoring their every word. Yet, candidates admit the real difficulty on the campaign trail is not the pressure-cooker life that comes with running for president. It's the lack of sleep they must endure in the process.

"I won't remember Iowans," Mitt Romney commented in Altoona. His wife, Ann, corrected him. What Romney meant to say was, "I'll never forget Iowans." In Iowa City, Hillary Rodham Clinton said, "We had three hundred people outside literally freezing to death." Literally, no one had died.

Commenting on the killing of Prime Minister Benazir Bhutto, Mike Huckabee offered his apologies. No, the sleep-deprived politician didn't kill the prime minister, despite his apology. His campaign staff came to his rescue and assured the American people that the candidate meant to offer his sympathies. Huckabee later admitted that the pressures of the campaign had made it impossible for him to get more than four hours of sleep per night.

President Barack Obama said ten thousand lives were lost when tornadoes ripped through Kansas. The actual death count was twelve. Obama blamed his overstatement on fatigue.

- **Get Treated for Obstructive Sleep Apnea**

Obstructive sleep apnea, a serious and potentially fatal disorder, affects approximately 10 percent of the adult population. Snoring, daytime fatigue, witnessed apnea (cessation of respiration for more than ten seconds), morning headaches, dry throat, and waking up gasping for air are common features of this disorder, which is being increasingly recognized as a formidable enemy of corporate America.

Sleep apnea prevents a person from reaching deep, restorative stages of sleep, making the person grumpy, irritable, nervous, forgetful, inattentive, and tired. It also increases the risk of stroke, heart attack, and early death because of the nightly struggle to breathe, which causes frequent elevation of blood pressure and sustained drop in blood oxygen level, while simultaneously increasing the oxygen consumption of the heart muscles. Untreated, sleep apnea increases the risk of motor vehicular and industrial accidents.

Take the STOP questionnaire to determine your risk for obstructive sleep apnea:

S—Do you **snore** loudly?

T—Do you often feel **tired**, fatigued, or sleepy during daytime?

O—Has anyone **observed** you stop breathing during sleep?

P—Do you have or are you being treated for high blood **pressure**?

If you answered yes to two or more of these questions, then you are at high risk for obstructive sleep apnea and should talk to your doctor.

To get an accurate diagnosis, you will need an overnight sleep study in a sleep lab where your respirations, oxygen level, heart rate, EKG, leg movements, and sleep stages will be monitored all night long without using needles. The commonest and most successful treatment includes wearing a mask hooked to a machine, called continuous positive airway pressure (CPAP), which acts as a pneumatic splint and prevents your throat from collapsing at night. The other options are weight reduction, oral appliance (a customized denture that keeps your lower jaw pulled forward), and ENT surgery.

It is extremely rewarding to be treated for sleep apnea. Patients have told me:

- "Doc, I did not know how sleepy I was until I started wearing a CPAP."
- "A hazy screen has been lifted off from my face."
- "I thought it was all stress and aging, but now I feel young again."
- "I am thinking clearer. I am planning better. I am getting more done at work and home."
- "I have so much energy that I don't know what to do with it."
- "My blood pressure is better; my sugars are better controlled."

- "I should have done this a long time ago."

If you suspect you have sleep apnea, please talk to your doctor. It will give you new life. If you need additional information, please visit my website (www.md4lungs.com) or watch my videos at www.youtube.com/yjpatel.

Eliminate Bad Sleep Habits

Poor sleep hygiene robs you of your deep sleep, makes your sleep nonrestorative, and thereby reduces your return on the investment of your time. This is a case of an iatrogenic, or self-inflicted, injury, which, as explained previously, discipline, dedication, and persistence can prevent. Please follow those good sleep habits you learned in the section on sleep hygiene with discipline and passion.

At some point in their lives, more than a hundred million people complain about difficulty falling asleep, staying asleep, or both. The economic burden of insomnia is humongous, with estimates running to tens of billions of dollars every year. In *Macbeth*, Shakespeare wrote, "Uneasy lies the head that wears the crown." Why can't a leader sleep? What can a leader do? What about sleeping pills? When should you see a sleep doctor? We will try to answer those questions in the following pages.

- **Eliminate Insomnia of Interpersonal Conflict**

One of the most common causes of insomnia in the workplace or in the family is interpersonal conflict. Interpersonal conflict is defined as an expressed struggle between at least two interdependent parties who perceive incompatible goals, scarce resources, and interference from the other party in achieving their goals. There are several causes of conflict. The most common ones are differences between people, needs, power, perceptions, principles and values, emotions and feelings, and internal problems and conflicts within a person.

Interpersonal conflict is everywhere today: conflicts between workers and supervisors, manufacturers and suppliers, two different departments, yourself and the CEO, mother and daughter, husband and wife, and so forth. The cost of all this interpersonal conflict, while difficult to measure, is nevertheless incredibly high. Interpersonal conflict is at the heart of war, for example. It is at the heart of domestic violence, road rage, and hate crimes.

In the business world, interpersonal conflict has a tremendous negative impact on productivity, morale, employee turnover, and workplace violence. In schools, interpersonal conflict often erupts into violence and even death. Medical researchers have found direct links between interpersonal conflict and disease; psychologists have found similar links between interpersonal conflict and mental health.

Insomnia is a common symptom of interpersonal conflict. So what can we do? Given the fact that the world in which we live is literally filled with interpersonal conflict, it's obvious we can't always avoid it. How then do we manage it? When it comes to interpersonal conflict, here are some options you may want to consider: flight, fight, or unite. The choice is yours.

Flight means you can walk away. Interpersonal conflict can't occur if only one person is involved. It always takes two. To walk away is to ignore the conflict, even if someone is being physically threatening to you. Walking away sends a strong message that you simply want to avoid the conflict, at least for the present. The other individual may interpret your action in a variety of ways, however, and this may actually escalate the conflict.

Choosing to fight is rarely the wisest choice. Even the simplest interpersonal conflict will escalate if you choose to psychologically or physically back your opponent into a corner and act threatening. And violence always escalates into more violence.

The best way to deal with interpersonal conflict is by uniting with those who want to engage in conflict in order to solve differences cooperatively. Talking through differences using respectful language and unthreatening body language can resolve most any conflict.

While major conflicts may require professional third-party intervention, the parties involved can resolve most interpersonal conflicts. Make it a point to resolve them. You'll feel better, and you'll sleep better.

Workplace stress is one of the commonest causes of insomnia. The following are a few pearls to help you manage stress successfully:

- Learn how to manage your time. Many people are stressed because they have trouble completing tasks on time. Look at your schedule and set your priorities.
- Learn how to deal with conflicts. When handling a difficult situation, keep your cool. When tensions are elevated, stress results.
- Learn to fit exercise into your daily routine. Exercise is a great way to relieve stress, so make sure you find time to get moving.
- Learn to eat healthy. Stop eating junk food for meals and snacks, and start eating healthy foods. Your body will cope with stress a lot easier. Reach for a piece of fruit instead of that bag of chips.
- Learn how to express your emotions. Talking to a friend or coworker about your feelings is a great way to combat stress. Don't keep your feelings bottled up.
- Learn the importance of a good night's sleep. Make sure you find time in your busy schedule to make it happen.
- Learn to have a positive attitude.

- **Sleep Soundly Even during Excitement**

Suppose that the innovative new product your team has been working on is ready for the big launch, which will open up new markets, increase your market share, put your company in the lead, and skyrocket your stock price. Prelaunch testing and research have all been positive. Popular media have given rave reviews, and they are covering the launch like the first iPhone launch. Your colleagues and your suppliers are all optimistic and excited about the new product. Can you turn off the adrenaline at bedtime? Can you shut off your mind when you put your head on the pillow? Can you sleep well during these times?

Here is another scenario: You have had a productive and very satisfying day at work. You are relaxing with your spouse. The kids are doing their homework. Then you get a text message from your star performer: "Sorry, I have decided to move on. I have accepted a job at another company." You knew this might happen, but you did not expect it so soon and at a time when things were going so well for the company and for your star employee. You have been through this before. It does give you an opportunity to find someone with a different skill set, but in the short run, it increases your workload. "I can handle that too. I'm not worried about this. I have built this company from scratch. I can tough it out until we can find someone good," you tell yourself. That night, you do not sleep well. The next morning, you wake up achy and tired.

Can you prevent this? Can you uncover anxiety when it is underneath the surface? And then can you successfully detach yourself from the troubles? Can you sleep well no matter what? You will have to, if you want to maximize your leadership during these exciting times. The following are a few helpful pearls[21] for those exciting or anxious times:

[21] Use these pearls for a similar challenge in your personal and your family life.

- Assign ten o'clock at night to six o'clock in the morning as sacred time, reserved for resting and recharging instead of planning and worrying.
- Get rid of all work-related material from your bedroom, including your laptop and smartphone.
- Continue your relaxing bedtime ritual: shower, relaxing reading, cookies and milk, and meditation, per your preference.
- Read your favorite lines from the Bible or any other religious book to calm your nerves.
- Turn off the lights and go to sleep.

Sweet dreams!

If you continue to have problems sleeping during exciting times, talk to your physician about using a mild sleep aid. This will prevent mounting sleep debt and, more important, prevent formation of an unhealthy conditioned reflex, which can perpetuate insomnia.

o Eliminate Anxiety about Falling Sleep

Psychophysiological (learned) insomnia refers to continued difficulty falling asleep, even after the initial stressor is long gone. The whole experience of going to bed reminds us of the difficulties we had during those stressful days. We dread going to bed. We are anxious and therefore more awake when we try to go to bed. We keep on worrying about the impact this will have on our life the next day. Recognize it. Learn self-relaxation. Progressive muscle relaxation is an easy-to-learn and immensely useful technique. Reassure yourself that one or two bad nights are not going to paralyze your executive abilities.

Learn and follow the suggestions for sound sleep discussed earlier.

In this section, we learned how to measure our sleep debt using the Epworth Sleepiness Scale. We also learned the deleterious effect of sleep debt on our executive function. Then we discussed common causes of sleep debt and what we can do about them. In the next section, we will learn to lead well during a major event or a tremendous opportunity, when sleep debt is unavoidable. Females[22] *in leadership position will find this section particularly helpful.*

---

22 I believe homemakers too can benefit from the advice given in this section as they are the leaders of their family.

Section V

Lead Well Despite Sleep Debt

- Monitor Your Alertness
- Follow the LAMP (Leader's Alertness Maximization Plan)
- Eliminate Midafternoon Madness
- Regain Your Evenings
- Be Happy Despite Sleep Debt
- Collaborate and Create Even When Tired
- Eliminate Irrational Fears
- Control Your Mirror Neurons
- Develop and Use Super Neurons
- Maximize Your Emotional Intelligence
- Remember Poor Sleep Impairs Your IQ
- Manage Information Well
- Use Your Spiritual Strength
- Dream Big Even When Sleepy
- Reverse Ability-Ambition Gap

- **Monitor Your Alertness**

As sleep debt increases, so does sleepiness. How can you fight this drowsiness when you cannot pay off your sleep debt because of the enormous challenges at work or at home? How can you maximize your alertness when sleep deprived? First, you will have to learn to monitor your alertness using Patel's Alertness Sleepiness Scale (PASS). To be able to live a rich and full life, you will need to be at a ten all day.

Patel's Alertness Sleepiness Scale (PASS)	
Feeling active, vital, alert, or wide awake	10
Functioning at high levels, but not at peak Able to concentrate	8
Awake but relaxed Responsive but not fully alert	6
Somewhat foggy Let down	4
Foggy Losing interest in remaining awake Slowed down	2
Sleepy, woozy, fighting sleep Prefer to lie down	0

- **Follow the LAMP (Leader's Alertness Maximization Plan)**

All day, and certainly during critical moments, measure and monitor your alertness using PASS. The surest and most natural cure for a low PASS is sleep, but what do you do when you cannot get sufficient sleep because of a hectic schedule and unavoidable demands? You can use the LAMP (Leader's Alertness Maximization Plan) to regain your alertness and thereby your leadership. Going against the might of Mother Nature, you can summon the help of these seven friends and design a LAMP applicable to your situation:

1. Physical exertion
2. PREM nap
3. Bright light
4. Caffeine
5. Smart snacking
6. Massage
7. Faith (my all-time favorite)

Also, beware of the formidable foe in alcohol when faced with insufficient sleep and long days.

1. Physical Exertion

Earlier, we discussed the importance of regular exercise on REM sleep and, hence, on alertness and the executive function. Here we discuss the role of physical activity in improving alertness when sleep deprived.

- **Deskercise for Deep Sleep**

On average, executives spend seven and a half hours per day sitting: in meetings, at their desks, in an automobile, or in boardrooms. Our bodies do not like staying still for long periods. That much sitting causes tension to build. Muscles become tight, and joints become stiff. Alertness starts declining the longer you stay still. One way to prevent these otherwise inevitable results of physical inactivity is to "deskercise" every hour.

Deskercising will help you reduce muscle tension and stress, while also helping you preserve the flexibility, strength, and muscle tone you already have. The following are some simple deskercising techniques to try:

- Wrist muscle stretch: Most executives spend a good deal of time in front of a computer. Computers have become essential tools in the management of business. However, with this increased use of computers, executives are becoming more susceptible to carpal tunnel syndrome, an ailment that used to be the exclusive domain of secretaries and other office workers who used typewriters and word processors most of the working day. Carpal tunnel is a painful wrist problem produced by repetitive motion. When working at the computer, stop occasionally and deskercise using the wrist muscle stretch: Slowly stretch your wrist muscles by using a full range of motion. Joints that have become sore and stiff because of repetitive-motion activity will respond to slow stretches. Don't risk pulling a muscle by attempting the stretch rapidly; get the full benefit by doing the stretch slowly. Not only will this give you a well-deserved break, it will go a long way toward preventing carpal tunnel syndrome.
- Pectoral stretch: This is an easy stretch you can do at your desk. Simply clasp your hands behind your head, and slowly move your shoulders and elbows back. Repeat this a few times. It is a great way to stretch your pectoral and chest muscles.

- Wrist flexion: Using your left palm, gently apply force to the right hand, causing the right wrist to stretch toward the underside of the right arm. Hold it there for five seconds and then release and repeat on the left hand. Repeat the exercise five times.
- Wrist hyperextension: Using the left palm, slowly apply force to bend the right hand backward. Hold it there for five seconds and then release and repeat to the left hand. Repeat the exercise five times.
- Sitting bend: In a sitting position, with your feet flat on the floor, your knees about ten inches apart, and hands at your sides, bend over as far comfortable with your hands reaching toward the floor. Hold the position for five seconds and then slowly pull yourself back into a sitting position while tightening your abdominal muscles. Repeat four times. This exercise stretches your lower back muscles and hamstrings.
- Vertical stretches: Vertical stretches provide an excellent way to reduce tension and activate all your major muscle groups. With your feet shoulder-width apart, lift yourself upward on your toes and extend your arms over your head. Reach each hand as high as possible for about seven seconds and then relax. Repeat four times.

- **Get Up and Walk Around**

Sitting too long can have several negative effects. It puts stress on the lower back and can lead to muscle atrophy and diminished flexibility. It's important to get up and walk around often. A ten-minute walk around the office is excellent. But, when that's not possible, shorter walks to the water cooler, filing cabinet, or restroom are better than nothing. Even when you're involved in meetings, seminars, or workshops, get up at least once every twenty minutes and move around. You'll feel better, you'll be healthier, and you'll sleep better.

In addition to physical exertion, use other key elements of a LAMP to maximize your alertness. Following are some tips for doing so:

2. **Take a PREM nap.** It can improve alertness for three hours. Studies have shown that a fifteen-minute nap can improve alertness and last for almost three hours. For specifics about PREM naps, refer to a discussion of it in section I.

3. **Get a relaxing massage**. Massage, especially when combined with a PREM nap, can improve alertness because it relieves muscle aches, back pain, headaches, burning in the eyes, and other distracting physical symptoms caused by sleep deprivation. Untreated, these symptoms can drag down your energy level and your alertness.
4. **Consume caffeine judiciously.** Caffeine has alerting properties, but it continues acting for twenty-four hours, so a cup of coffee consumed at one o'clock in the afternoon is still in your bloodstream at midnight when your brain is trying to get into REM sleep. For this reason, caffeine should not be used indiscriminately, but rather as a medicine, at the right dosage, at the right time, and for the right reason. The surest indication for caffeine is driving when sleep deprived. Then it can be lifesaving.

5. **Look at the light often.** Bright light has tremendous alerting influence. Use this to your advantage. Sit facing the window. During long meetings in the boardroom, look up at light often. Especially on cloudy days, put a bright-light lamp behind your desktop while working. Every fifteen minutes, turn off the PowerPoint presentation and turn on the lights.
6. **Snack smartly.** Small protein snacks every two to three hours will maintain your energy and alertness; on the other hand, eating a large starchy meal will degrade your alertness. Grilled fish or chicken is fine. Avoid rice, pasta, and dessert.
7. **Seek spiritual support.** This has helped me the most during my post-call days in the clinic. Going from one exam room to the next, I would look up and ask for divine help. "Give me energy, my Lord, to serve my patients well."

Here are a few additional pearls, which would help you achieve maximal alertness.

- **Avoid alcohol.** Even the legal limit of alcohol will impair your leadership when you are sleep deprived. When there is still work to be done, avoid even a small glass of wine or a beer. Resist that temptation.

- **Eliminate Midafternoon Mistakes**

Most mammalian species have a second sleep period during the daytime because of the midafternoon dip in alertness. This dip in the middle of the working day causes a decline in executive output and, more important, creates an environment conducive to disastrous mistakes. The following graph depicts the number of sleep-related accidents and their time of occurrence. Please note the steep increase in accidents between one and three in the afternoon.

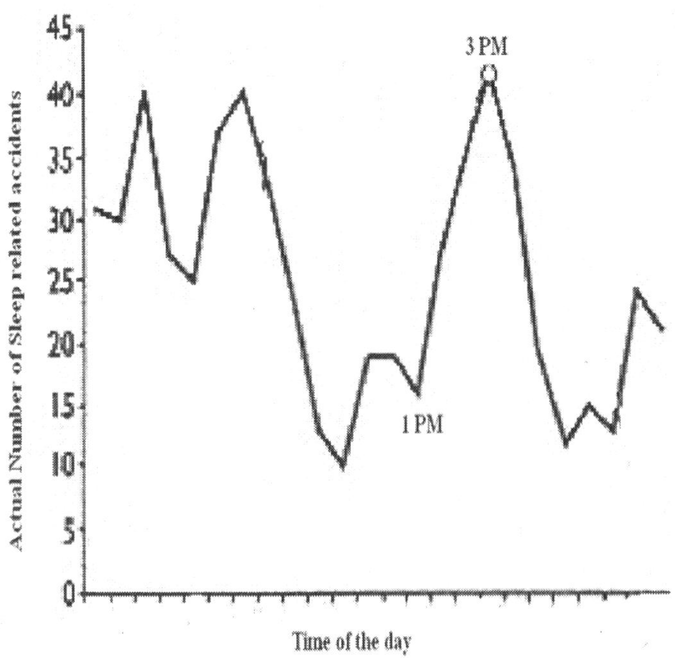

Incidence of sleep-related vehicle accidents (n=606) by hour of day. *BMJ* 1995;310:565 Sleep-related vehicle accidents. J. A. Horne, professor, L. A. Reyner, research associate, Sleep Research Laboratory, Department of Human Sciences, Loughborough University, Leicestershire.

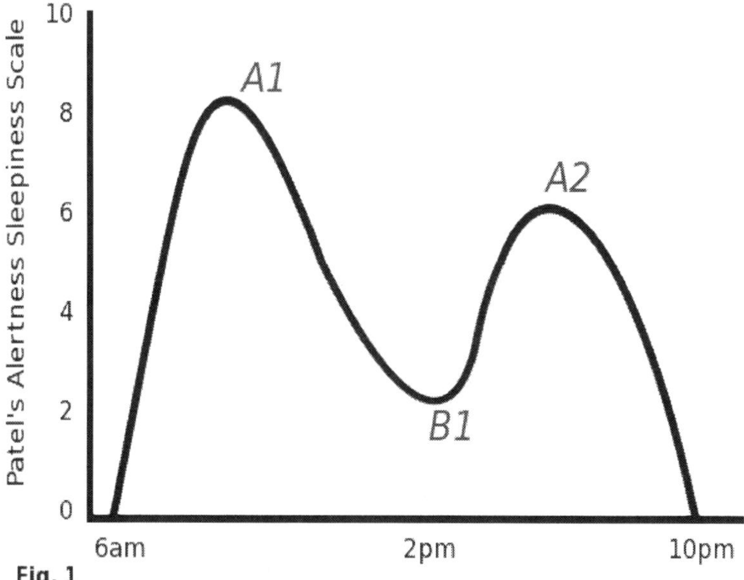

The above graph highlights circadian fluctuations in our alertness during a typical day at work. Remember that at B1, you may blow up on your teenager. Intensive-care-unit rounds, board meetings, financial planning, and important negotiations should be done at A1.

No matter what industry you work in, you will identify with the midafternoon madness that seems to take place among leaders and managers everywhere. Complacency and chaos tend to rear their ugly heads soon after lunch. Keep these tips in mind to help you get through the midafternoon madness:

- Take a fifteen-minute PREM nap in the early afternoon. It will go a long way toward improving your performance as a leader.

- Make sure you find a way to fit in thirty minutes of exercise each and every day, including weekends. When you do, you will drastically improve the quality of your sleep, which will ultimately make you a stronger and wiser leader.
- Eat a hearty breakfast, but a light lunch. If you avoid carbohydrates at lunch, you will not feel sluggish at the next afternoon meeting. Your brain will be able to think more clearly and handle crucial decision-making duties.
- If you receive an irate telephone call or e-mail, stop and count to ten. Avoid the temptation to fire back with anger and resentment. If you are sleep deprived, the situation will only become worse. Never let an e-mail or a telephone call get you so mad that you react like a child. Count to ten, take a walk around the block, or do whatever you need to do so you can respond with a clear and level head.
- When midafternoon madness strikes, do not make any long-term commitments.

- If at all possible, avoid scheduling any important meetings around the two o'clock time slot. Most people are so groggy from overeating or drinking at lunch that they will not be able to pay attention to important details.
- Keep moving. Get up and do some physical activity for at least ten to twenty minutes. It will help to keep the blood circulating and clear your head at the same time.
- Follow your Leader's Alertness Maximization Plan (LAMP).
- Avoid task–ability mismatch. Beware of doing high-complexity tasks or making important decisions in the afternoon.

- **Regain Your Evenings**

Early-morning leaders run out of energy and end up underperforming in the evening meetings. Here are some tips you can use to regain your evenings:

- Plan and take a ten- to fifteen-minute PREM nap prior to three o'clock. This will give you a second wind in the evening.

- Avoid heavy meals in the evening.
- An evening walk or exercise can be alerting. Get up and start walking as soon as you notice lethargy creeping in.
- It breaks my heart to tell you that even a glass of wine can drag your alertness down. Resist that temptation, especially if you have an important event in the evening.
- Caffeine can be alerting, but it will rob you of your deep sleep. It is best to avoid it.

If you follow the above recommendations, you can achieve rectangular alertness.

Rectangular Alertness

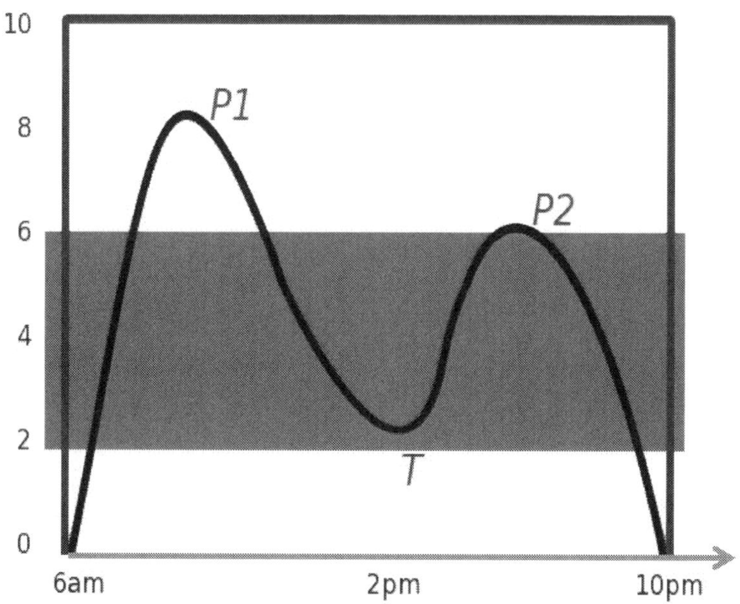

In the above graph, P1 and P2 refer to the peak alertness we experience in a typical day, while T refers to the trough in our alertness felt midafternoon. By using the techniques discussed in this book, we can achieve rectangular alertness and feel maximally alert all day long.

So far in this section, we have discussed suboptimal alertness and countermeasures we can employ to improve alertness and thereby achieve rectangular alertness. Now we will discuss sleep deprivation's deleterious effects on emotional intelligence and countermeasures we can employ to overcome them. Here is a list of those deleterious effects.

1. When sleep deprived, we are unable to accurately recognize emotions. Unfortunately, negative emotions are more readily recognized than positive ones.
2. Studies have shown decreased subjective rating of happiness by sleep-deprived people.
3. Our overactive fear center exaggerates our fear and anger when sleep deprived.
4. Sleep deprivation impairs our social interaction and learning because of perception fatigue.
5. A study from the Neuroscience Lab in Singapore showed that when sleep deprived, we are reactive and not proactive.
6. Nervousness, irritability, and grumpiness hurt our teamwork.
7. Impaired self-evaluation resulting from sleep deprivation makes us unaware of our deficits.
8. Studies have also shown reduced motivation, increased risk taking, and indecisiveness when faced with an ethical dilemma.

Here are a few pearls to help you eliminate these deleterious effects.

- **Be Happy Despite Sleep Debt**

Happy people lead a richer life, but it is difficult, if not impossible, to maintain a pleasant demeanor and optimism when sleep deprived. Chronically running on insufficient sleep, we are grumpy, irritable, pessimistic, unpleasant, parochial, lethargic, complacent, and, hence, ineffective as a leader. This worsens when we encounter an unexpected challenge that unfortunately deepens our sleep deprivation.

Let's look more closely at the cause of impaired emotional intelligence and the countermeasures you can employ to overcome that impairment and be a happy, optimistic, enthusiastic, charismatic, productive, and influential leader. Remember, positive emotions lead to positive life.

- **Collaborate and Create Even When Tired**

When you watch a scary movie, your amygdala, a primitive reptilian structure, is activated, but the prefrontal cortex informs it that this is not an actual threat. The prefrontal cortex calms down the amygdala in a split second, so we do not act on our fears. But when sleep deprived, if the amygdala perceives danger, it goes into overactive mode, unchecked by logical reasoning from a now-underactive prefrontal cortex, and it releases a large amount of adrenaline hormone, which sets the leader in fight-or-flight mode, as opposed to collaborate-and-create mode.

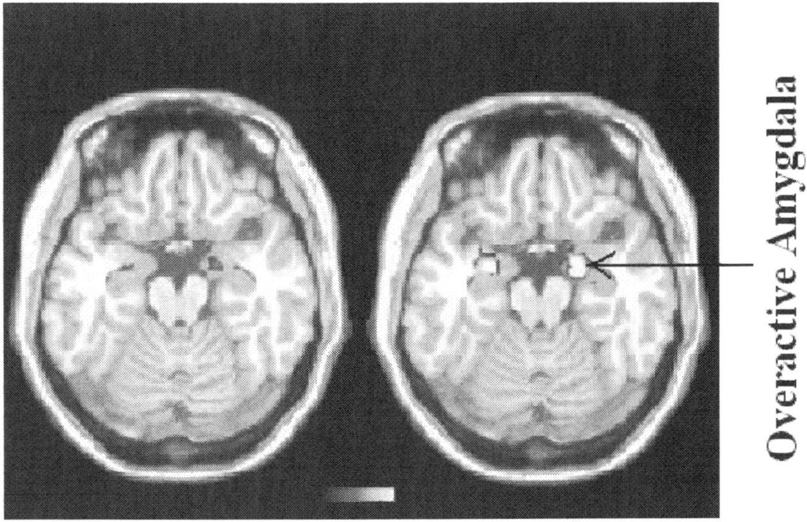

Brain scans showing amygdala responses to increasingly negative emotional stimuli in the control groups (left) and the sleep-deprivation group (right). (From *Current Biology* 17 (20). The human emotional brain without sleep: a prefrontal amygdala disconnect. Seung-Schik Yoo, Ninad Gujar, Peter Hu, Ferenc A. Jolesz, and Matthew P. Walker.)

For a moment, consider what this means, especially for those females in leadership roles where others' economic, social, and physical well-being lies in the balance. A leader whose prefrontal cortex has been temporarily shut down could suddenly face an emergency situation where clear thinking and exceptional problem-solving skills are a must. What price would society pay for that particular leader's lack of sleep?

- **Eliminate Irrational Fears.**

Monkeys are born with a paralyzing fear of snakes. But interestingly enough, when their amygdala is surgically destroyed, monkeys eat these snakes alive. Sleep deprivation makes the amygdala overactive, which further exaggerates our irrational fears.

How common are these fears? During my Executive MBA program, at the beginning of our semester-long marketing elective, professor Phillip Raskin gave us five minutes to think about our biggest fear, write it on a piece of paper, and give it to him. He filed those papers in a folder and began his class. As the semester progressed, we got extremely busy with assignments and deadlines, and completely forgot about the informal study the professor had done of our fears. We were shocked and surprised when he shared the results in our last class. Forty-two out of forty-six students had written fear of failure as their biggest fear. Can you imagine the impact of this on our goal setting[23]? It can make a difference between Jeff Bezos staying in Manhattan as an investment banker or starting Amazon.com.

---

[23] This is the reason Facebook's corporate office has "What would you do today if you weren't afraid?" written on its walls.

Imagine this fear getting further exaggerated from an overactive amygdala, the fear center. I remember going to our hospital strategy retreats after my seventy-two-hour ICU calls. Forget about suggesting and setting big, hairy, audacious goals; I was even afraid to set goals within our core competency. Be cognizant of truncated goal setting as a result of irrational fears.

Sleep deprivation also weakens one's ability to integrate emotion and cognition to guide moral judgments. A study showed that, when faced with an ethical dilemma, a sleep-deprived leader would have significant indecisiveness in making a decision in favor of the greater good, an effect that emotional intelligence partially neutralizes.

- **Control Your Mirror Neurons**

Our brain is made up of a hundred billion neurons (nerve cells), each of which is connected to thousands of neurons through synaptic connections. Located in the frontal cortex, a small subset of neurons called motor command neurons fires when the person performs a specific action or observes someone else perform the same action. For example, when you try to open a bottle of wine or observe a friend trying to open a bottle of wine, the same set of neurons in your frontal cortex is activated. These are called mirror neurons.

Christian Keysers and his colleagues at the Social Brain Lab have shown that similar mirror neurons also exist for emotions. This discovery has great practical implications for leaders, because these neurons, once activated, can transmit both negative and positive emotions across the organization, making it a huge collection of neurons separated only by skin!

When exposed to our colleagues' negative emotions, our mirror neurons are activated in microseconds. What happens next has profound implications at the departmental level, corporate level, and national level. In the presence of sleep deprivation, with an overactive amygdala and an inactive executive center, a chain reaction starts, which recruits more and more neurons, leading to a viral epidemic of negative emotions.

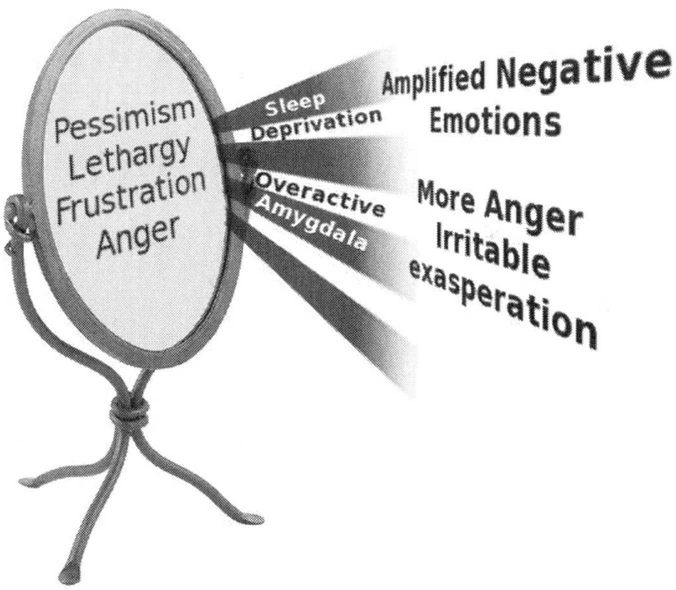

Colleagues' and friends' negative emotions activate our mirror neurons. An overactive amygdala amplifies these negative emotions, which rapidly spread across the organization.

- **Develop and Use Superneurons**

How can you prevent such an epidemic of negative emotions? Even when faced with negative emotions expressed by followers, a well-rested female with a well-regulated amygdala and hyper-vigilant executive center will recruit neurons with positive emotions. Here is the billion-dollar question, though: can we transform negative emotions in the presence of sleep deprivation, overactive fear center, and underactive executive center?

Yes, we can, by developing unconditional empathy toward everyone involved. The neurons responsible for such transformation are called superneurons. By nurturing and using these superneurons, a leader can rapidly spread a viral epidemic of optimism, innovation, ethics, integrity, exuberance, service, sacrifice, humility, euphoria, and success across a large organization—using mirror neurons. This is how Jeff Bezos sustained momentum and spread optimism at Amazon.com despite negative cash flow year after year. This is how Mahatma Gandhi spread his message of nonviolence, one neuron at a time, to three hundred fifty million illiterate Indians in the absence of a free press.

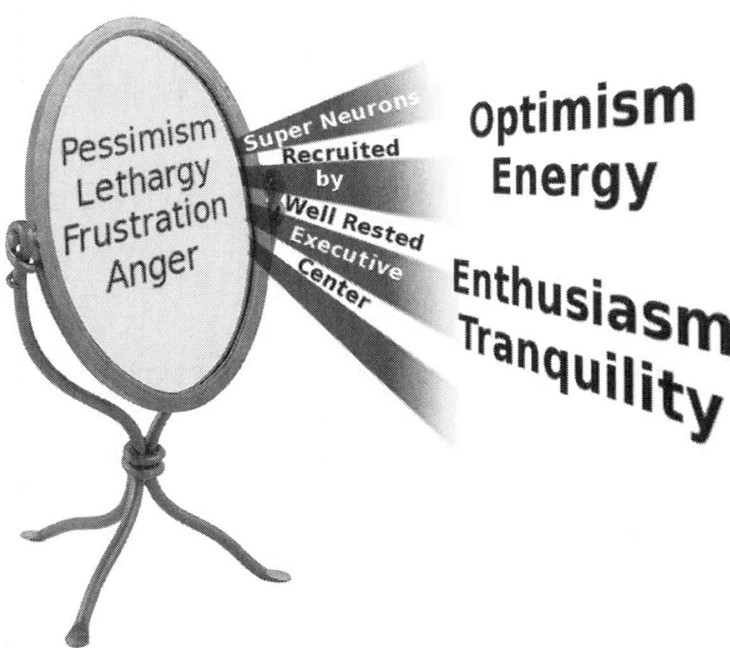

Colleagues' lethargy and pessimism reflexly activate our mirror neurons, but a well-rested prefrontal cortex activates superneurons and transforms these negative emotions into positive ones. Because of these superneurons, leaders transform pessimism, lethargy, frustration, and anger into optimism, energy, enthusiasm, and tranquility.

- **Maximize Your Emotional Intelligence**

If you answer five simple questions, you will know what your emotional intelligence score is.

1. Can you recognize your emotions?
2. Can you manage your emotions?
3. Can you recognize others' emotions?
4. Can you manage others' emotions?
5. Are your social skills at their best?

Give yourself two points for each yes answer and zero points for each no answer. The first two questions measure self-management. The next two measure interpersonal intelligence. The last one measures your social skills. Let's look at them one by one.

- **Recognize your emotions.** When sleep deprived, we are sometimes too tired to care about recognizing and describing our emotions, but it can help us greatly if we can learn to accurately recognize our emotions. Look at the following list. Circle the words that represent how you are feeling. Accurately recognizing your emotions helps you manage them.

Embarrassed	Overwhelmed	Afraid	Excited
Fearful	Proud	Awful	Friendly
Brave	Furious	Sad	Calm
Scared	Cheerful	Gloomy	Serious
Happy	Stressed	Comfortable	Ignored
Cruel	Interested	Tense	Curious
Thrilled	Depressed	Lonely	Uncomfortable
Mad	Worried	Elated	Nervous
Angry	Fantastic	Pleasant	Annoyed
Relaxed	Bored	Frustrated	Relieved
Gentle	Safe	Caring	Generous
Clumsy	Guilty	Shy	Confused
Stubborn	Creative	Impatient	Surprised
Jealous	Thoughtful	Delighted	Joyful
Disappointed	Loving	Weary	Disgusted

- **Manage your emotions.** Once you have recognized and described your emotions, the next step is to learn to transform the negatives ones into positive emotions. The following steps can help you do that:
    - Diagnose emotions. Do not ignore them.
    - Try to find the cause. You are impatient because you want to finish the meeting, go home, and relax. Or you are upset because your colleague has not done what he had promised to do. Or you are anxious because the deal you thought you had sealed might not go through.
    - Seek support from your spouse. Remember, you have been through worse before.
    - Have faith. Do a one-sentence prayer. Forgive yourself and forgive others. Learn mindfulness meditation.
    - Sit straight and stand upright. An interesting study showed higher levels of testosterone and cortisol levels in participants who sat in a power posture than those who had slumped down in the chair.

  - Walk with a bounce, and talk with a smile. A fake bounce and fake smile light up the same neurons as a genuine bounce and genuine smile.

Once you go through these steps, circle your emotions again. Hopefully, you will see some positive emotions now.

- **Recognize others' emotions.** Sleep deprivation causes emotional agnosia, the inability to recognize others' emotions. To make matters worse, this selective agnosia makes us recognize negative emotions more readily than positive ones, resulting in pessimism and poor interpersonal communication when sleep deprived. How can we overcome this?
  - Gather intelligence about their emotional intelligence. Know the emotional makeup of the attendees beforehand.
  - Look them in the eyes. Remember, motor neurons fire when we watch others perform. Make it a habit, even when alert, to look into a person's eyes when talking and listening. Carry this habit forward, especially when sleep deprived.
  - Listen more than you talk. Pause and perceive.

- Name those emotions. Use your newly acquired inventory of words. Find the right word from your memory to describe the emotions your colleague is going through.

- **Manage others' emotions.** Use the following tips to help you deal with others' emotions:
  - Acknowledge others' feelings. This can have a very calming effect on destructive emotions.
  - Even in the face of insults, accusations, delays, and failures, maintain your tranquility. Only by maintaining evenness of mind can you manage others' emotions successfully and become a problem solver, as opposed to a problem creator.
  - Find the root cause of the negative emotions, and explain your point politely and calmly.
  - Offer a break from intense work. Offer to go for a cup of decaf coffee or to talk about something not so contentious.
  - Practice, practice, and practice. Learn to manage emotions with enthusiasm and patience. Do it at every opportunity you get.

- **Maximize your social skills.** When we are sleepy, we are not at our best in social interactions. We are too sleepy to care, talk, or connect. How can you connect even when tired? The following are a few helpful tips:
  - Smile and share happiness.
  - Learn the big art of small talk.
  - Express genuine interest in others' lives and interests.
  - Relax and enjoy. If you *are* relaxed, you will appear relaxed.
  - Look in their eyes when talking.
  - Keep your arms open rather than crossed and closed. Positive body language is extremely important in your interactions with other people.
  - Be humble and polite.
  - Leverage your positive personality traits.
  - Learn to pause and share your thoughts. Share your opinion clearly and politely. Be open to others' opinions.
  - Identify what makes you uncomfortable, and then plan, practice, and enjoy.

- Record in your smartphone what their interests and hobbies are.
- Be patient. Improving your social skills is a slow process.

Even when tired, female leaders form lasting bonds.

The following are steps to happy life even when sleep deprived:

- Exude contagious enthusiasm and optimism. It will spread rapidly across the organization.
- Recognize that a smile is your savior. Humor and happiness stabilize a leader's intellect. Smile often. Stay close to people with positive demeanors.
- Recognize that pause is your partner. Pause before answering. Save emotional e-mails in the drafts folder and send them the next morning. If it is a complicated issue or a vital one, sleep on it.
- Do not dwell on the unpleasant aspect of your work.
- Pray often. When on the go, read a line from the Bible or other spiritual book.
- Replace fear and anger with faith and empathy through mental discipline.

- Avoid irritability. Take a walk, talk to your spouse, nap, meditate, exercise, and play. Beware of delicate situations that can exaggerate irritability. Tactfully avoid them or live through them quietly.
- Listen to the lazy one on your team or in your life.
- Look for collaboration and creativity.
- Set the goals high.

Thus far in this section, we have learned about rectangular alertness and emotional intelligence. Remember, happy females have bigger networks and richer lives. Next, we will learn about successful information management even in the presence of sleep deprivation.

"Because there are three classes of intellects: one which comprehends by itself; another which appreciates what others comprehend; and a third which neither comprehends by itself nor by the showing of others; the first is the most excellent, the second is good, the third is useless." —Niccolò Machiavelli

o Remember Poor Sleep Impairs Your IQ

As summarized in the following list, sleep deprivation adversely affects every facet of information management.

1. When sleep deprived, we have a short attention span and suffer from easy distractibility.
2. Studies have shown that our working memory,[24] procedural memory, and declarative memory[25] are also impaired.
3. We are unable to consolidate and then retrieve memory when sleep deprived.
4. We are also unable to incorporate new information into our decision-making.

---

[24] It enables us to remember several pieces of information while we try to use it to solve a problem or carry out a task.

[25] A memory that can be consciously discussed, or declared.

5. An interesting study gave participants sets of words like "hazy, cloudy, and dark." After sleep deprivation, they were asked if "black" was one of the words. Surprisingly, sleep-deprived individuals confidently gave wrong answers! Could this be the reason why honest people sometimes lie with confidence?
6. Sleep deprivation also leads to rigid thinking and cognitive fixation (ignoring facts that do not agree with our diagnosis).
7. Sleep deprivation causes a lack of verbal fluency.
8. In a study using master planner activity, sleep debt caused production misjudgment and loss of profitability.
9. Sleep deprivation also impairs creative problem solving and causes perseverance errors (trying an unsuccessful solution repeatedly).

Air traffic control had cleared the airplane for takeoff on runway 22, which is 7,003 feet long and equipped with high-intensity runway lights; however, the crew mistakenly taxied onto runway 26, which is 3,500 feet long and unlighted, and attempted to take off. The airplane ran off the end of runway 26, impacted the airport perimeter fence and trees, and crashed. Of the forty-seven passengers and three crewmembers on board the airplane, forty-nine were killed, and one received serious injuries.

During its investigation of this accident, the safety board learned the air traffic controller who cleared the accident airplane for takeoff had worked a shift from six thirty in the morning to twelve thirty in the afternoon the day before the accident and then returned nine hours later to work the accident shift from eleven thirty until the time of the accident at seven minutes after six the next morning. The controller stated that his only sleep in the twenty-four hours before the accident was a two-hour nap the previous afternoon between the two shifts.

- **Manage Information Well**

The following pearls will help you manage information effectively and avoid similar disaster:

- Solicit novel ideas and suggestions. Methods should be flexible; goals may not be.
- Avoid internal distractions. Train your mind to stay focused on the task at hand. One pointed mind will achieve more at a majestic pace than a distracted mind at a frantic pace.
- Minimize external distractions. Discourage your colleagues from making distracting comments. Politely bring them back to the task at hand.
- Compile vital information in one location, as opposed to keeping it in various folders in various locations.
- Write, draw, write, draw, and remember. Verbal memory is more affected than visual memory.
- Prepare, write, and rehearse. Speak slowly and clearly. Avoid tongue twisters and long sentences.
- Scrutinize, verify, and dissect the data. At retrieval, sleep deprivation causes false memories.

- Seek simplicity. Bravely and mercilessly weed out unnecessary detail.
- Sleep on it if possible. REM sleep causes crazy creativity. Or listen to the lazy one on your team, or consult your spouse, parents, mentor, or well-rested buddy.
- Do not try failed solutions repeatedly.

We just talked about how you can successfully manage information in the face of sleep debt. Now, we will briefly talk about how you can maintain your faith and dream big even when running on insufficient sleep.

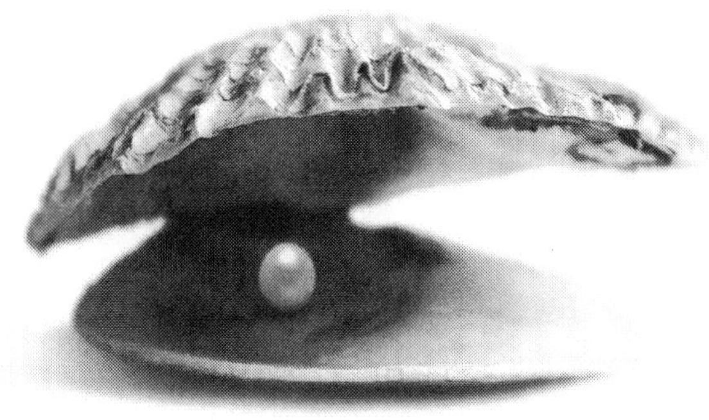

Use Your Spiritual Strength

Sleep deprivation adversely affects our faith and makes us ignore and, hence, underutilize our spiritual strength. We need to be cognizant of this handicap and find a routine such as prayer, regular meditation, frequent visits to our church, or continual consultation with our spiritual guru. Then we should stick to it, especially when setting our goals in life, planning our career, or facing adversity on our journey. Remember, faith sustains leadership.

Sleep deprivation's adverse effect on faith unfortunately gets worse with aging. Have you noticed how younger leaders demonstrate unbridled enthusiasm, set audacious goals, carry crazy creativity, and possess bold ideas? For most of us, aging, reality, and past work experiences moderate these qualities. Leaders, on the other hand, continue to nourish, nurture, and grow such enthusiasm and creativity throughout their long careers because of their deep faith. This unshakable faith annihilates their amygdala's irrational fear and helps them reach their true potential.

The corporate world today demands revolutionary ideas, actions, and results from its female leaders. The only way a leader can deliver on this demand is by harnessing and utilizing spiritual strength. Deep faith and spiritual strength will help us see a future we can shape together for the advancement of the human race. Without faith and spiritual strength, Mahatma Gandhi could not have successfully sold his idea of nonviolence to three hundred million Indians, most of them illiterate, despite state-controlled media. When faced with insurmountable obstacles while working on our vision, a deep faith and spiritual strength will propel us past the problems.

- **Dream Big Even When Sleepy**

The University of Notre Dame began on the bitterly cold afternoon of November 26, 1842, when a twenty-eight-year-old French priest, the Reverend Edward Sorin, and seven companions took possession of 524 snow-covered acres in the Indiana mission fields. In 1879, when a disastrous fire destroyed the main building, which housed virtually the entire university, Father Sorin vowed to rebuild the university and continue its growth.

"I came here as a young man and dreamed of building a great university in honor of Our Lady," he said. "But I built it too small, and she had to burn it to the ground to make the point. So, tomorrow, as soon as the bricks cool, we will rebuild it, bigger and better than ever."

That campus has grown from 524 acres in 1842 to 1,250 acres and 140 buildings. The University of Notre Dame today is a leading academic institution in the world. This would not have been possible without Father Sorin's unshakable faith and deep spirituality.

- **Reverse Ability-Ambition Gap**

Sheryl Sandberg, chief operating officer of Facebook, speaking at Columbia University in New York, shared a striking observation that female leaders' ambitions were much lower than their ability unlike their male counterparts, whose ambitions far exceeded their ability. Sufficient sleep and unshakable faith can help reverse this mismatch. And when working on insufficient sleep, please make a conscious effort to reverse this mismatch.

Concluding Comments

You work hard both at home and at work, where you fight male dominance every day. You shoulder more than your share of family responsibilities, while suffering from insufficient sleep during premenstrual syndrome, menstruation, pregnancy, lactation, menopause, and postmenopause. This sleep debt gets worse when faced with new challenges or opportunities at home or at work. I still remember my ICU calls that were thirty-six hours and sometimes seventy-two hours long, which I suffered through from 1989 to 2009. During that time my leadership and my life passed by, which I did not realize at the time. I have combined that unique experience with the latest medical research to come up with a framework that will empower you to regain that lost leadership and life itself. I want you to be better prepared than I was at handling crises both at home and at work, and more important, at enjoying work and cherishing this wonderful gift called life.

Remember that we are here on this beautiful earth for only a finite amount of time. The only way we can squeeze maximum life out of each moment is by maximizing our alertness, even during stressful periods. I know this is an uphill battle, but with patience, perseverance, practice, and faith, you will learn to excel and enjoy despite unavoidable sleep debt.

Guard your sleep like you guard your life. And when you cannot get sufficient sleep because of stress at home or at work, use the LAMP (Leader's Alertness Maximization Plan) to maximize alertness. Leverage this alertness to maximize your emotional intelligence and informational intelligence. Add selflessness and spirituality to this mix, and you will maximize your God-given potential.

God Bless You. Best Wishes. Keep in Touch.

Appendix A

Behavior change takes time, patience, and persistence. Follow me on http://www.twitter.com/yatinjpatel and receive my tweets about sleep disorders, sound sleep tips, sleep news, leadership, and life. Here are a few of my past tweets:

- Pleasant and perpetual perception is a prerequisite to consistent excellence.
- Sleep on your back and avoid facial wrinkles.
- As I dream 2night, my Lord, take me to enchanted corners of every galaxy.
- Dreams are a testament to brain's limitless imagination. Dream well 2night.
- As I sleep, my Lord, replace hatred from my subconscious with faith and love.
- As I sleep, Lord, fill up my vast subconscious with hope, happiness, joy, & bliss. And then wake me up with highest level of consciousness.
- We are what we think. Let us have noble thoughts today.

- Humor and happiness stabilize a leader's intellect. Keep me happy today, Lord.
- Help me spread contagious enthusiasm & optimism across the organization.
- Wakefulness is the way to life. Help me serve from the highest level of wakefulness.
- Help me serve humanity with unshakable faith, empathy, and enthusiasm.
- Help me enjoy every moment today.
- Be my energy today.
- Give me the strength to carry on.
- Infuse noble thoughts from every direction.
- Can problems lead to internal peace and harmony instead of turbulence and frustration?
- You shall find unending joy, when you expel lust, hatred, and fear from your mind.
- Peace is always at the center of incessant activity. Find it.
- Each moment contains a beautiful life within. Cherish it.

- Dream big tonight, dream even bigger tomorrow. Good night my friends.
- Find #peace amid incessant activity this week. Good night friends.
- Pray on the pillow to wake up with vigor and vitality. Good night friends.
- As I sleep, my Lord, please replace fear and hatred from every neuron with faith and love. Good night to all.
- Purge your mind of negative #emotions. They get amplified during REM #sleep. Good night friends.
- In your dreams, move with love even among the unloving. Good night from Goshen.
- Poor sleep stimulates brain's fear center Amygdala, while our faith annihilates it. Maintain faith today at work!
- Sound sleep will lead to world peace. Sleep well, my friends.
- Uncertainty is awesome! Embrace it. Enjoy it.
- There is no wrong place or posture to take a PREM power nap!

Appendix B

Suggested Books

The Harvard Medical School Guide to a Good Night's Sleep (Harvard Medical School Guides) by Lawrence Epstein and Steven Mardon (paperback)

The Promise of Sleep: A Pioneer in Sleep Medicine Explores the Vital Connection Between Health, Happiness, and a Good Night's Sleep by William C. Dement and Christopher Vaughan (paperback, 2000)

Emotional Intelligence: 10th Anniversary Edition; Why It Can Matter More Than IQ by Daniel Goleman

Say Good Night to Insomnia by Gregg D. Jacobs (paperback, 2009)

The Insomnia Workbook: A Comprehensive Guide to Getting the Sleep You Need by Stephanie Silberman and Charles Morin (paperback, 2009)

No More Sleepless Nights by Peter Hauri and Shirley Linde (paperback, 1996)

Restful Insomnia: How to Get the Benefits of Sleep Even When You Can't by Sondra Kornblatt and Teresa E. Jacobs, MD (paperback, 2010)

I Can Make You Sleep: Overcome Insomnia Forever and Get the Best Rest of Your Life! by Paul McKenna (hardcover and CD, 2009)

Cognitive Behavioral Treatment of Insomnia: A Session-by-Session Guide by Michael L. Perlis, Carla Jungquist, Michael T. Smith, and Donn Posner (paperback, 2008)

Power Sleep: The Revolutionary Program That Prepares Your Mind for Peak Performance by James B. Maas, Megan L. Wherry, David J. Axelrod, and Barbara R. Hogan (paperback, 1998)

Take a Nap! Change Your Life by Sara Mednick and Mark Ehrman (paperback, 2006)

Permission to Nap: Taking Time to Restore Your Spirit by Jill Murphy Long (paperback, 2002)

Sleep to be Sexy, Smart, and Slim by Ellen Michaud (2008)

A Woman's Guide to Sleep: Guaranteed Solutions for a Good Night's Rest by Joyce Walsleben and Rita Baron-Faust (paperback, 2001)

Sleep Deprived No More: From Pregnancy to Early Motherhood—Helping You and Your Baby Sleep Through the Night by Jodi A. Mindell (paperback, 2007)

The Well-Rested Woman: 60 Soothing Suggestions for Getting a Good Night's Sleep by Janet Kinosian (paperback, 2002)

Suggested Websites

www.sleepfoundation.org

National Sleep Foundation

www.nhlbi.nih.gov/about/ncsdr

National Center on Sleep Disorders Research, National Institutes of Health

About Me

Born in India, in a small university town, where my father ran a printing and publishing business, I went to medical college there and then came to the United States in 1987. I did my internal medicine residency (1989–1992) at Mount Sinai Hospital in New York, where I was also the chief resident. After finishing pulmonary and sleep-medicine fellowship in 1994, I founded the Center for Sleep Studies and started my pulmonary and sleep-medicine practice at Sneeze & Snooze Clinic in Goshen, Indiana. I also served as the director of pulmonary medicine at the Indiana University Health Goshen Hospital. I am a senior fellow at the American College of Chest Physicians and American Academy of Sleep Medicine, where I am an active member of the sleep deprivation subcommittee.

In 2002, I started the public awareness campaign "Stay Awake, Drive Safe," aimed at eliminating drowsy driving-related accidents through educational events at schools, colleges, and highway rest plazas.

In 2008, I graduated magna cum laude from the Executive MBA program, Mendoza College of Business, at the University of Notre Dame. I consult with organizations of various sizes, educate their executives on the importance of sleep, and help sleep-deprived executives excel despite insufficient sleep. I conduct seminars, "Supreme Leadership through Sound Sleep" and "AEI∞ Model of Supreme Leadership."

I am a frequent contributor on WNDU (NBC), WSTV (FOX), WNIT (PBS), and B100 (radio), promoting sleep. My hobbies include nature, meditation, philosophy, wine, and cooking. I live in Goshen, Indiana, with my wife, Dipti, my daughters, Priyata and Pooja, and my son, Parth. I can be reached at md4sleep@gmail.com. Find me and connect with me on Facebook, Twitter, LinkedIn, and Google+.

Thank you. God bless you. Keep in touch.

Price: 99 cents (eBook) and 9 dollars (paperback)

Profits from the sale of this book and from my consulting work will go toward supporting a global initiative, the F.E.M.A.L.E. (Food, Education, Medicines, And Love for Everyone) Ashram, aimed at changing the world by educating one neuron at a time through innovative intervention using the Internet and other media.